INNER
HEALING
FOR MEN

INNER HEALING
FOR MEN

ARTHUR L. MACKEY, JR.

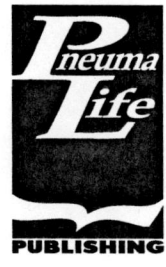

PUBLISHING

INNER HEALING
FOR MEN

ARTHUR L. MACKEY, JR.

Copyright © 2001 Arthur L. Mackey, Jr. - ISBN 1-56229-123-8

Pneuma Life Publishing, Inc.
4423 Forbes Blvd.
Lanham, Maryland 20706
301-577-4052
http://www.pneumalife.com

Printed in the United States of America 1 3 5 7 9 10 8 6 4 2

CONTENTS

1

The Masculine Cry for Wholeness - Inner Healing for Men

Today there is a universal cry that echoes deep within the hearts of men. It is a brutal, bone-chilling cry for inner healing. Yes, inner healing from the vicious pains and wounds of our past that literally haunt our present efforts. It threatens the very existence of our future endeavors as men in drastic need of meaning.

Way beneath our phony facade of invincible masculinity, all men are actually fragile creatures controlled by the curiosity of the unknown, whether positive or negative. Without the guidance of Jesus Christ we are mere ordinary men. Only God Himself has the power to put the jagged-edged pieces of our battered, broken, and bruised existence back together again.

We need to move to the next level; we need to come out of the stagnant stage we are in spiritually, socially, or economically and move to the next stage of maturity and responsibility as sons, brothers, fathers, husbands, friends, and mentors.

Inner healing for men begins with you and me. Inner healing begins with the admission that we need help from above to move to the next level.

Just one touch from the Master's hand can inspire a deeply discouraged and despondent man to discover his divine destiny and catch God's vision of victory. Yes, inner healing for men requires a purely divine touch of destiny from the Master's nail-scarred hands upon our tortured souls. Only He can help us face our own daily demons of self-destruction.

These daily demons of self-destruction prevent us from moving to the next level. They teach us to ignore our wives, our children, and all forms of responsibility. God wants to start with the very heart of man and teach us individually and collectively how to get those demons cast out. We can do that only by using the name of Jesus, and through true personal responsibility rooted and grounded in the life-changing blood of the crucified Lamb of God.

The joy of the Lord is the most potent source of inner strength for a wounded man in search of real meaning and purpose in life. In his classic book, *Jesus Man of Joy*, Sherwood Eliot Wirt, founding editor of *Decision* magazine, writes that the "The secret of Jesus was—and is—His inner joy."[1]

A WOUNDED SPIRIT

The writer of the Book of Proverbs accurately declares in chapter 18:14, *"The spirit of a man will sustain his infirmity; but a wounded spirit who can bear?"* In the original Hebrew text, the word "wounded" is *naka* and means to be afflicted, broken, smitten, and stricken. Can you hear the constant cries of wounded, hurting men, many of whom were wounded in the homes of their own friends?

Regrettably, this constant cry for inner healing is not always verbalized. Too often this silent cry creates inner turmoil too difficult to face alone. But the heavenly Father yearns to strengthen our wounded hearts. Ephesians 3:14-16: *"For this cause I bow my knees unto the Father of our Lord Jesus Christ, Of whom the whole family in heaven and earth is named, That he-would grant you, according to the riches of his glory, to be strengthened by his Spirit in the inner man."*

Being around a man with a broken spirit can be one of the most depressing experiences in life. A man in need of inner healing has dreams of destiny that are now dormant; his visions of victory are now vague thoughts of better days. A man in need of inner healing has had his hope toward God crushed by the reality of life's ups and downs.

Inner healing is needed for men who have lost all hope. They are candidates for the Creator's creative workshop called "inner healing for men." These are men who have seen their promised rainbow turn into a dismal, dark sky. Men with money and no integrity. Men with integrity and no financial resources. Men on the verge of divorce. Men who have a lover on the side. Men who have problems communicating and accepting the truth. These men, who are living in the night season of life, need inner healing.

THE NIGHT SEASON

This night season may have been going on for a long time. There have been too many nights of cruising around looking for bars and hangout joints, too many nights of spending the family's money in all the wrong places. There have been too many nights out of the will of God, because such a man is angry with God, angry at the world, and angry with himself.

Inner healing for men may not occur through serving Jesus only as the Savior of our souls, but rather in having an intimate, open, and honest relationship with God. We need to make Him the Lord over all the public and private areas of our lives. God is calling on men to forsake the foolish mess of being phony macho men who need no help and no God. A phony, superficial, grandiose man is a man who gives himself all the glory and constantly ignores his own dire need for inner healing and essential wholeness.

The prolific poet, J. G. Holland, said it this way:

God, give us men!

A time like this demands strong minds, great hearts, true faith and ready hands;

Men whom the lust of office does not kill;

Men whom the spoils of office cannot buy;

Men who possess opinions and a will;

Men who have honor;

Men who will not lie;

Men who can stand before a demagogue and damn his treacherous flatteries without winking;

Tall men, sun-crowned, who live above the fog in public duty and in private thinking.

It is only when a good man's footsteps are divinely orchestrated, ordained, and ordered by the Lord that man can muster the inner strength to overcome the fact that he has failed, faltered, and fallen from God's grace. A good man, who truly wants to walk in the warning, anointing, and admonition of the Almighty, will run back to God's everlasting arms. Only then will he find fulfillment, after his fall, that only the Father, Son, and Holy Spirit can give.

Psalm 37:23-25 says, *"The steps of a good man are ordered by the Lord: and he delighteth in his way. Though he fall, he shall not be utterly cast down: for the Lord upholdeth him with his hand. I have been young, and now am old; yet have I not seen the righteous forsaken, nor his seed begging bread."*

THE FIRST ADAM

The first man, Adam, is the first example of a real man—designed by God--who was in drastic need of inner healing. Genesis 2:7 states: *"And the Lord God formed man of the dust of the ground, and breathed into his nostrils the breath of life; and man became a living Soul."*

God put Adam in charge of the Garden of Eden, a perfect place to live. One night God put Adam to sleep, took a spare rib from his side and made Adam a beautiful woman, Eve.

Genesis 2:21-25 put it this way: "*And the Lord God caused a deep sleep to fall upon Adam, and he slept: and he took one of his ribs, and closed up the flesh instead thereof; And the rib, which the Lord God had taken from man, made he a woman, and brought her unto the man.*

"*And Adam said, This is now bone of my bones, and flesh of my flesh: she shall be called Woman, because she was taken out of Man. Therefore shall a man leave his father and his mother, and shall cleave unto his wife: and they shall be one flesh. And they were both naked, the man and his wife, and were not ashamed.*"

Because of the couple's lack of communication, Eve listened to the serpent instead of her husband and ate some fruit that God had forbidden them to eat. Eve also convinced Adam to eat the forbidden fruit; God held Adam accountable for this disobedience that caused the fall of man. After Adam, the first man, disobeyed God, all of mankind was in need of inner healing for a sin-sick soul.

Like many of us, Adam tried to hide from God. But God asked Adam in Genesis 3:9, "Where art thou?" God knew exactly where Adam and Eve were: hiding in their nakedness in the trees of the garden. God was really asking Adam, "Where are you spiritually?" God was letting Adam know that he was now in need of inner healing for his wounded soul.

Edwin Louis Cole declares in his book, *On Becoming a Real Man* that, "Real manhood cannot be found in just a moment's emotional outburst. Neither is real manhood found in the image of physical prowess and handsomeness. Nor in personality, talent, intelligence, performance, or profession. Real manhood is found within the heart of a man, the 'inner man,' his moral character, the 'real man' that exudes beyond all external devices for the rest of the world to see."[2]

Even Jesus Christ Himself, the last Adam, a Man above all men, the Savior of all mankind, emphasized the importance of inner healing for the brokenhearted. In Luke 4:18-19, Jesus declared that *"The Spirit of the Lord is upon me, because he hath anointed me to preach the gospel to the poor; he hath sent me to heal the brokenhearted, to preach deliverance to the captives, and recovering of sight to the blind, to set at liberty them that are bruised, To preach the acceptable year of the Lord."*

IRON SHARPENS IRON

Inner healing for men is a timely subject. God is calling on men to share testimonies concerning the daily obstacles, trials, and tribulations of real manhood. Proverbs 27:17 says, *"Iron sharpeneth iron; so a man sharpeneth the countenance of his friend."* A man of purpose who gets close to God and prayerfully exchanges positive and pertinent life-changing information with other men can brighten up and sharpen the countenance and future of other men.

Proverbs 20:5 says, *"Counsel in the heart of a man is like deep water; but a man of understanding will draw it out."* A man of understanding will pull out the best in you. A man of understanding will draw out the dormant, stagnant, and still waters that run deep within the masculine souls of men searching for true inner healing and essential wholeness.

A man of understanding who is truly anointed by God with a fresh word of wisdom can inspire you to pull up, draw out, and deal with real hard-core issues of life from the deepest waters of your masculine soul that your subconscious has purposely made you ignore for years.

The Bible clearly sets the standard for men of destiny to sharpen one another with a simple concept that works: older men who dream dreams must invest in younger men who will see visions. Joel 2:28 states: *"And it shall come to pass afterward, that I will pour out my spirit upon all flesh, and your sons and daughters shall prophesy, your old men shall dream dreams, your young men shall see visions."*

God is calling older and more mature Christian men to be role models and mentors—like Moses and Elijah—to the younger Christian men, the visionary Joshua and Elisha generation of today.

That is why Proverbs 4:23 stresses: *"Keep thy heart with all diligence; for out of it are the issues of life."* As older and younger men—destiny dreamers and visionaries—we must sharpen one another by sharing the importance of guarding our affections, desires, passions, and lust for the lively, because they impact every area of our lives positively or negatively, according to the current status of character deeply embedded within our hearts.

Uncontrolled affections can ruin a man's dream and his vision. For where our treasure is, there our heart will be also.

Gordon MacDonald states within his book, *When Men Think Private Thoughts*, that "Now if manhood is merely a matter of testosterone and the possession of male genitals, there is no problem. But probably every male knows in his soul that there is a problem, for manhood is more that a hormonal or an anatomical matter. Manhood is a way of thinking, being, and functioning. It is a social statement of who I am and who others think me to be. It is an issue of role, what place do I have in the community, and how am I valued in the position?"[3]

The spirit of man is the candle of the Lord; God has ordained that the light of His love will shine through the spirits of mankind. When the spirit of a man is sustained, preserved, and guarded by the Holy Spirit, that man has the power to overcome any affliction, infirmity, temptation, or test that storms the gates of his masculine soul.

Proverbs 20:27 supports this statement: *"The spirit of man is the candle of the Lord, searching all the inward parts of the belly."*

A SECOND CHANCE AND A NEW HEART

God wants to provide a second chance and a new heart to wounded men who are truly in need of and want their inner healing. He wants to reach men who were made in the image of God, but have lost their direction. God wants to make you a brand new man right now, my brother.

In the classic book, *The Measure of A Man* by the late civil rights leader Dr. Martin Luther King, Jr., declared, "So I say to you, seek God and discover him and make him a power in your life. Without him all of our efforts turn to ashes and our sunrises into darkest nights. Without him, life is a meaningless drama with the decisive scenes missing. But with him we are able to rise from the fatigue of despair to the buoyancy of hope. With him we are able to rise from the midnight of desperation to the day break of joy. Saint Augustine was right—we are made for God and we will be restless until we find rest in Him."[4]

The Father still yearns to perform open heart surgery or even a heart transplant on your tortured spirit and make you a new man of destiny, a man transformed one day at a time through the positive and progressive renewal of your mind with the Word of God.

2

MEN OF DESTINY

The Lord wants to recruit real men with real problems, real heartaches, and real pains, who will truly seek His face, and not only His mighty hand. Psalm 27:8 says, "*When thou saidst, seek ye my face; my heart said unto thee, Thy face, Lord, will I seek.*" Seek His face. Don't seek worldly success, for true biblical success—the wisdom to walk effectively in the affairs of real life—is the result and byproduct of actually seeking the Lord's face.

In the book, *Let Go of Whatever Makes You Stop,* motivational speaker John Mason states, "The man who has no direction is the slave of his circumstances. The poorest man is not he who is without a cent, but he who is without purpose."[5]

True worship is a key component of the Christian life because it creates an atmosphere for inner healing and essential wholeness. True worship requires total surrender to God from the very depths of our inner man, our human spirit, the candle of the Lord. Inner healing for men can only be found by ultimately tapping into God's everlasting reservoir of living water, the Holy Spirit, a spiritual source of inner strength far greater than our own male egos.

A man's ego cannot eliminate, erase, or eradicate the pains of a problematic past or the frustrations of a fatalistic future. But the anointing of the Holy Spirit can destroy our yoke of bondage, the negative fate that Satan designed for our personal demise and defeat, with a positive and progressive plan of divine destiny that God the father personally ordained for us.

RISE UP, O MEN OF GOD

"Rise up, O men of God! Have done with lesser things; Give heart and mind and soul and strength to serve the King of Kings.

Rise up, O men of God! His Kingdom tarries long; Bring in the day of brotherhood, and end the night of wrong.

Lift high the cross of Christ! Tread where His feet have trod; as brothers of the son of man rise up, O men of God!" ("Rise Up, O Men Of God") [6]

The men of destiny who wholeheartedly seek to embrace the sovereignty of God's guidance, instead of wasting precious time by walking in the ways of the wicked, will find peace—the essence of true success in the midst of the storm—despite any personal inner struggles against the daily attacks of Satan.

Psalm 1:1-5 declares, "*Blessed is the man that walketh not in the counsel of the ungodly, nor standeth in the way of sinners, nor sitteth in the seat of the scornful. But his delight is in the law of the Lord, and in his law doth he meditate day and night. And he shall be like a tree planted by the rivers of water, that bringeth forth his fruit in his season; his leaf also shall not wither; and whatsoever he doeth shall prosper.*

"*The ungodly are not so: but are like the chaff which the wind driveth away. Therefore the ungodly shall not stand in the judgment, nor sinners in the congregation of the righteous. For the Lord knoweth the way of the righteous: but the way of the ungodly shall perish.*"

INNER HEALING IN THE MIDST OF THE STORM

Psalm 37:37 declares, "*Mark the perfect man, and behold the up-right: for the end of that man is peace.*" To me, inner healing means receiving the peace of God that passes all understanding and em-powers us to go through, deal with, and overcome the real-life per-sonal struggles, storms, and frustrations of the moment.

Philippians 4:7 boldly declares, "*And the peace of God, which passeth all understanding, shall keep your hearts and minds through Christ Jesus.*" Yes, a place of peace in the midst of major family problems and financial crisis.

Isaiah 26:3 states: "*Thou wilt keep him in perfect peace, whose mind is stayed on thee: because he trusteth in thee.*" God will make a place of peace to get your life back together again. A place where—in the midst of troubled marriages, gruesome separations, deadly divorces, and hopelessness—you can find peace.

Philippians 4:8-9 says, "*Finally, brethren, whatsoever things are true, whatsoever things are honest, whatsoever things are just, whatso-ever things are pure, whatsoever things are lovely, whatsoever things are of good report; if there be any virtue, and if there be any praise, think on these things. Those things, which ye have both learned, and received, and heard, and seen in me, do; and the God of peace shall be with you.*"

Yes, a place of peace in the midst of broken promises and for-gotten dreams. Jesus Christ said it this way, as recorded in John 14:27 (NKJV): "*Peace I leave with you, My peace I give to you; not as the world gives do I give to you. Let not your heart be troubled, neither let it be afraid.*" Yes, a place of peace that transformed mere ordi-nary men who were dirty, old liars from every imaginable walk of life into promise seekers well on the road to becoming promise keepers through the grace of God.

REPENTANCE

Mere ordinary men truly need inner healing to be totally trans-formed through time into extraordinary men of divine destiny. Only then can they learn to address the thunderous storms of life through true humility, the power of prayer, seeking God's face, and responding to our Father's clarion call for real repentance. (See 2 Chronicles 7:14.)

Then and only then will our heavenly Father hear our cry of real repentance, forgive our sins, and heal the land of our masculine insecurities.

Anthropologist David Gilmore comes to an extremely interesting conclusion in his thought-provoking book *Manhood in the Making*. His book is the very first cross-cultural case study of manhood defined as an attained goal or an achieved societal status. Through his intense research Gilmore comes to the surprising conclusion that real manhood embraces the notion of nurturing as a valid expression of mature masculinity.

Gilmore states in his research that, "Again and again we find that 'real' men are those who give more that they take; they serve others. Real men are generous, even to a fault, like the Mehinaku fisherman, the Samburu cattle herder, or the Sambria or Dodoth big man. Non-men are often those stigmatized as stingy and unproductive. Manhood therefore is also a nurturing concept, if we define that term as giving, subventing, or other-directed."[7]

Inner healing for men is a God-ordained process pertaining to real repentance. It provides mere men with a profound sense of purpose to overcome the sinister strongholds of Satan, both individually and collectively.

Second Corinthians 10:4 states: *"For the weapons of our warfare are not carnal, but mighty through God to the pulling down of strongholds..."* The preordained purpose of God Almighty is to enhance, empower, and enrich the lives of men—regardless of our circumstances, our job status, our racial heritage, and whether we live in the slums or in a fancy penthouse. As men, we are mandated by the Father to pull down satanic strongholds that push us out of the perfect will of God.

We learn to pull down these satanic strongholds—sins of habit and weaknesses—with the spiritual weapons of our warfare by trusting in God's mighty power to help us resist our temptation or repent of our transgression in the time of trouble.

This universal cry of inner healing and essential wholeness for wounded men was expressed with great pain and anguish when the influential King of Israel, David, pleaded for forgiveness of his own personal sins. He had fallen from God's favor, due to his own premeditated adultery with Bathsheba and his murder of her husband, Uriah. David purposely placed Uriah in the front lines of battle to be slain, brutally murdered for the king's own lustful convenience.

Second Samuel 12:1-7a states: *"And the Lord sent Nathan unto David, And he came unto him, and said unto him, There were two men in one city; the one rich, and the other poor. The rich man had exceeding many flocks and herds; But the poor man had nothing, save one little ewe lamb, which he had bought and nourished up: and it grew up together with him, and with his children; it did eat of his own meat, and drank of his own cup, and lay in his bosom, and was unto him as a daughter. And there came a traveler unto the rich man, and he spared to take of his own flock and of his herd, to dress for the wayfaring man that was come unto him; but took the poor man's lamb, and dressed it for the man that was come to him. And David's anger was greatly kindled against the man, and he said to Nathan, As the Lord liveth, the man that hath done this thing shall surely die: And he shall restore the lamb fourfold, because he did this thing, and because he had no pity. And Nathan said unto David, Thou art the man."*

After the powerfully anointed prophet Nathan confronted King David with his horrible sin against God and with his own personal weakness, David cried out to God in a critically important and powerfully anointed prayer of real repentance. It was from the depths of his own tortured soul. David truly pleaded with God for forgiveness, *"Create in me a clean heart, O God; and renew a right spirit within me. Cast me not away from thy presence; and take not thy Holy Spirit from me. Restore unto me the joy of my salvation; and uphold me with thy free spirit"* (Ps. 51:10-13).

God forgave David and gave him back the joy of his salvation. As men, we can also experience the magnificent power of God's forgiveness if we truly wait on the Lord in true repentance and humility. Psalm 40:1-3 says, *"I waited patiently for the Lord; and he inclined unto me, and he heard my cry. He brought me up also out of an horrible pit, out of the miry clay, and set my feet upon a rock, and established my goings. And he hath put a new song in my mouth, even praise unto our God: many shall see it, and fear, and shall trust in the Lord."*

The Man in the Glass

(Author Unknown)
When you get what you want in your struggle for self
And the world makes you king for a day,
Just go to a mirror and look at yourself
And see what that man has to say.

For it isn't your father or mother or wife
Whose judgment upon you must pass;
The fellow whose judgment counts the most in your life
Is the one staring back in the glass.

Some people might think you're a straight-shooting chum
And call you a wonderful guy.
But the man in the glass says you're only a bum
If you can't look him straight in the eye.

He's the fellow to please; never mind the rest,
For he's with you clear to the end.
And you have passed your most dangerous test
If the guy in the glass is your friend.

You may fool the whole world down the pathway of years
And get pats on your back as you pass.
But your final reward will be heartache and tears
If you've cheated THE MAN IN THE GLASS.

A MAN AFTER GOD'S OWN HEART

David's willingness to admit his transgressions against God through real repentance made him a man after God's own heart. David seriously sought the face of God—in many different situations—as the ultimate Source of inner healing for his tortured soul that was cast down in severe depression.

David was not playing with God. David truly wanted his soul to be right with God. Psalm 42:1-5 says, *"As the hart panteth after the water brooks, so panteth my soul after thee, O God. My soul thirsteth for God, for the living God: when shall I come and appear before God? My tears have been my meat day and night, while they continually say unto me, Where is thy God?*

"When I remember these things, I pour out my soul in me: for I had gone with the multitude, I went with them to the house of God, with the voice of joy and praise, with a multitude that kept holy day. Why art thou cast down, O my soul? and why art thou disquieted in me? hope thou in God: for I shall yet praise Him for the help of his countenance."

Although no sin is too big for God to forgive, His forgiveness does not eradicate sin's natural consequences. The natural consequences of sin remain a reality in spite of God's forgiveness. For example, according to 2 Samuel 2:15-19, David and Bathsheba's first child died as a direct result of their sin against God.

It does not pay to play with God. Don't think for a minute that you can just enjoy your sin tonight and repent tomorrow. Throughout his life, David had to constantly encourage himself in the Lord in one situation after another, even before he knew Bathsheba, to survive his inner turmoil in life-threatening situations and receive his inner healing.

First Samuel 30:6 states: *"And David was greatly distressed; for the people spoke of stoning him, because the soul of all the people was grieved; every man for his sons and his daughters: but David encouraged himself in the Lord his God."*

Sometimes people will be ready to kill you because of your faults, but remember that God has a plan for your life. Don't even think of giving up. Repent and get right with God regardless of whether or not you win the respect of people. Repent and ask God to teach you responsibility. Repent and ask God to send you a strong, godly spiritual mentor who will show you how to be a real Christian man—not only in word, but also in deed.

Ask God to teach you to be a better father. Ask God to walk with you day by day and teach you how to treat a woman and how to love a wife as Christ loved the church and gave His very life for it. Ephesians 5:25-28 says, "*Husbands, love your wives, even as Christ also loved the church, and gave himself for it; That he might sanctify and cleanse it with the washing of water by the word, That he might present it to himself a glorious church, not having spot, or wrinkle, or any such thing; but that it should be holy and without blemish. So ought men to love their wives as their own bodies. He that loveth his wife loveth himself.*"

THE MARRIAGE MASSAGE MINISTRY

This might sound silly to some folks, but I must be honest. One of the ways I find the truth of inner healing in the natural sense is by giving my wife a massage. Brenda asks me for a good massage just about every single day that the Lord gives us. My wife is a mental health worker and works with mentally ill patients. After a long day of being on her feet, she needs a good massage. I've discovered true inner healing and essential wholeness in a purely natural sense—with tremendous spiritual overtones—by giving my wife a massage. It makes me realize that if Jesus Christ, my risen Lord and Savior, could endure the brutal torture, agony, and pain of the cross at Calvary and give His own life for you and me, then I can at least give Brenda—my baby, my honey, my lover, my wife—a massage. I also help out in other practical ways in the raising of our three adorable children: Yolanda, Jordan, and Faith.

If Jesus Christ could die on the cross and rise again from the dead for our emancipation from the brutal bondage of sin and Satan, then it is not a crime for me to change a diaper or do some laundry when I can. If Jesus could die on the cross for me, then it is not a crime for me to talk to my wife and learn day by day how to effectively communicate with her. That is the least I can do, considering the enormous price that Jesus paid for His bride, the church.

3

CRYING OUT TO THE CREATOR

R eal men need to cry out to the Creator for inner healing and essential wholeness, no matter where they're at in life: the alley, the street corner, a war-torn community, the inner city, the ghetto, the suburbs, or a state-of-the-art office complex. God will respond to their cries by fanning the fresh flames of a revolutionary revival that will spread like wild fire in the lives of spiritually wounded men.

As men, we must learn to cry out to the Creator for personal and corporate revival like David did. As deep calling unto deep at the noise of God's refreshing waterspouts, so the waves and billows of His healing streams will flow over our tortured souls (see Ps. 42:7).

God wants to empower men with inner healing, for men of destiny should always pray and not faint. Too many men are fainting, falling, and failing their families because of a failure to wait on the Lord for guidance and direction. Before King David died, he told one of his sons— Solomon, who succeeded him as King—to be a man who walks in the way of the Lord.

Second Kings 1:1-3 says, *"Now the days of David drew nigh that he should die; and he charged Solomon his son, saying, I go the way of all the earth: be thou strong, therefore, and shew thyself a man; And keep the charge of the Lord thy God, to walk in his ways..."* When Solomon showed himself to be a man who reverenced God, God blessed him. But when Solomon did his own thing, he suffered with inner turmoil because of his own self-righteousness and self-indulgence."

When mere ordinary men wait on the Lord, God will grant a divine renewal of inner strength for facing life's journey. He'll bless them with a fresh sense of vigor and vitality. God desires to grant inner healing for men to be delivered from the lies of the past, present, and future. Psalm 40:4 boldly declares, *"Blessed is that man that maketh the Lord his trust, and respecteth not the proud, nor such as turn aside to lies."* A man needs inner healing to stop abusing his wife and children—verbally, mentally, physically, and economically. He needs inner healing to learn to love, nurture, and give his life for his wife.

Inner healing will enable us as fathers to spend quality time with our children and not try to buy their love with gifts that cannot father them. Steve Farrar stated in *Anchor in Man*, "Children obviously need food, clothing, shelter, and medical attention. But they need more! They need their father's love. They need their father's wisdom. They need their father's concern. They need their father's discipline. And the only way they are going to get those things is if they get something else. They need their father's time."

Ephesians 6:4 states: *"And ye fathers, provoke not your children to wrath: but bring them up in the nurture and admonition of the Lord."* Inner healing will enable us as fathers to hold our children in our arms, instill a sense of safety in their lives and tell them who they are. This will instill purpose and destiny in their spirit and soul.

Proverbs 20:7 states that *"The just man walketh in his integrity: his children are blessed after him."* Real manhood is not best expressed in the power to impregnate a woman, but rather in the power to be a responsible father and a positive male role model.

Josh McDowell writes in *The Father Connection* that the task of being a father is of critical importance and it has never been more so than in this day and age. A child's relationship with Dad is a decisive factor in the young man or woman's health development and happiness.[9] The last verse in the Old Testament, Malachi 4:6, declares, *"And he shall turn the heart of the fathers to the children, and the heart of the children to their fathers, lest I come and smite the earth with a curse."*

The Holy Spirit will provide deep inner healing to enhance, enlighten, enrich, and empower men. It will never emasculate the wounded souls of hurting men. God wants to give inner healing for men to be like:

- Abraham, a pioneer of faith in the midst of life's impossibilities.

- David, a man after God's own heart.

- Noah, who built an ark and walked in obedience to God.

- Daniel, able to sit in a lion's den of real-life situations and not be afraid because of God's protection.

- Joseph, trusting God to deliver him personally from the pit of despair, the time of temptation, and the prison.

- Nehemiah, rebuilding the broken-down walls of a war-torn community

- the apostle Paul and know God in the power of the resurrection and the fellowship of His suffering.

Inner healing to move to the next level and realize that God never gave up on any of these men in spite of their many faults. God will never give up on you!

TRANSFORMATION

If God can make a murderer into a totally transformed man seeking after God's own heart, a liar into a man of integrity and a father of faith, a drunk into a man of destiny, and a persecutor of the church into an anointed preacher of the gospel, then God can work a miracle in your life. He can move you to the next level in life and teach you how to live right. He can show you how to live an honest lifestyle of holiness before the Lord, who sees what we do at all times.

Most of all, God wants to grant inner healing so men can understand the seasons of God. So they can walk with Jesus, the Master of destiny, and be transformed into real men for all seasons who are seasoned with the salt of God's everlasting love. The Holy Spirit of God wants to care for, carry, and comfort wounded men who are hurting badly and crying out for inner healing and essential wholeness.

Inner healing for men takes on a fresh, new meaning for the masculine mind when men discover that not only does God want to save our souls from an eternal burning hell, but He also wants to discipline our masculine spirit, soul, and body to withstand the chaotic storms of life. He wants to teach us day by day how to handle the hardships that we experience as chosen soldiers in the army of the Lord.

THE MEASURE OF A MAN

(Author Unknown)
Not how did he die,
but how did he live? Not what did he gain,
but what did he give?

These are the units that measure a man is a man regardless of birth.
Not what was his station,
nor did he have heart,
but how did he play his God-given part?

Was he ever ready with a kind word of cheer to bring back a smile or to banish a tear?
Not what was his church,
not what was his creed,

but did he befriend those who were in need?

Not what did the sketch in the newspapers say,
BUT HOW MANY PEOPLE WERE SORRY WHEN HE
PASSED AWAY?
WHAT WILL PEOPLE SAY OF YOU?

TRUTHS FROM KING DAVID

In Psalm 22, King David, under the divine unction and anointing of the Holy Spirit, shares some profound truths concerning his own experience of inner healing. David was a man full of perplexing anguish, inner turmoil, and frustration with God. In the midst of his personal pain and miserable existence as a man in search of hope and inner healing, King David cried out these words of anguish in Psalm 22:1: "*My God, my God, why hast thou forsaken me? Why art thou so far from helping me, and from the words of my roaring?*"

Have you ever felt that God had forsaken you? I have. Scripture promises that God will never leave us nor forsake us. But it never promised that we would not feel forsaken and all alone, like a motherless child left on some old, dusty doorstep. Yes, even as men with a mission in life, we will sometimes feel forsaken and all alone.

It is in these personal moments when real men cry out, "Oh, my God," in their own private prayer closets amidst the pulsating pressure of the night seasons of life. It is in these personal moments that real men cry out in anguish to God in the night seasons of personal pain and private sin. It is in these very personal moments that real men are not at a loss for words. They are not silent, but are angry at God for the burdens they bear as men in need of meaning.

It is in these heated conversations with the Creator that real men must come to the realization that God is God. He is infinite and man is finite. God has all power and man has no power—without God. Like Jesus on Calvary's old, rugged cross of crucifix-

29

ion, King David knew that God would never forsake him, yet he felt alone. And that's OK, because sometimes a real man has to feel all alone in order to honestly search his own masculine heart and soul in such a compete way that he truly finds God's unlimited source of inner healing.

It was King David who wrote, in Psalm 37:25, "*I have been young, and now am old; yet have I not seen the righteous forsaken, nor his seed begging bread.*" It is only human to feel forsaken, but we discover God's eternal lifeline of inner healing and essential wholeness for real men when we realize that God is holy. He can make us whole by inhabiting our praise.

As a real man of integrity, Nehemiah, put it this way: "for this day is holy unto the Lord: neither be ye sorry; for the joy of the Lord is your strength." The realization that yes, God is real, even in the midst of our personal pain, allows real men to release their praise and worship to the Creator, who cares for men even in times of crisis and chaos. Our high praise and worship make the heart of God joyful, and the joy of the Lord is our strength. The joy of the Lord is our only real, lasting source of inner healing and essential wholeness."

So King David humbled himself before the mighty hand of God and said, in Psalm 22:6, "*But I am a worm, and no man: I am the scorn of men, and despised by the people.*" He discovered true inner healing by praising and worshipping God among his fellow believers. That is how God still wants men to find inner healing today—by praising, worshipping, and yielding our very lives by crying out from the depths of our souls, "Yes, Lord! Yes, to Your will, and yes, to Your way."

In essence, King David said, "I will praise God with my brothers, right in the midst of my mess and my loneliness. I will praise the name of the Lord with my brothers, right in the midst of my own personal pain, problems, and predicaments. I will magnify the name of the Lord among my brethren and get my inner healing. Psalm 22:22 says, "*I will declare thy name unto my brethren: in the midst of the congregation will I praise thee.*"

Something happens when real men see other men praising, worshipping, and yielding their lives to the Lord in the midst of their personal pain. Inner healing begins. We need to spread the word and share the message.

King David declared: "They shall come, and shall declare his righteousness unto a people that shall be born, that he hath done this." But before King David, the mighty man of war, could say that God had done this, and before Jesus Christ, the Savior of the world, could say on the cross, in a far greater sense, "It is finished," they both had to process their personal pain and find inner healing. It's an inner peace that only the Heavenly Father can give.

Inner healing and inner peace teach us that God hates our personal and private sin, but God does not hate us. God hated the sin of the world that Jesus carried for the redemption and salvation of mankind, and even Jesus felt forsaken and alone, but God knew exactly what He was doing.

Remember that before King David could make his bold declarations stated so eloquently in the Twenty-third Psalm, he had to process his pain through the power of praise and worship unto God, who delivered him and will deliver you. It was in this context of triumph over enduring personal pain that King David, the mighty man of war, wrote:

"The Lord is my shepherd; I shall not want. He maketh me to lie down in green pastures; he leadeth me beside the still waters. He restoreth my soul; he leadeth me in the paths of righteousness for his name's sake. Yea, though I walk through the valley of the shadow of death, I will fear no evil: for thou art with me; thy rod and thy staff they comfort me. Thou preparest a table before me in the presence of mine enemies: thou anointest my head with oil; my cup runneth over. Surely goodness and mercy shall follow me all the days of my life: and I will dwell in the house of the Lord for ever."

The late civil rights leader, Dr. Martin Luther King, Jr., expounded with great eloquence the true essence of inner healing for men when he wrote in *The Measure Of A Man:* "I don't know about you, but when I look at myself hard enough I don't feel like crying with the Pharisee, 'Lord, I thank thee that I am not like other men,' but I find myself crying out, 'Lord, be merciful unto me, a sinner.'" Humility is mandatory for real men to yearn for inner healing from the divine touch of the Master's hand. [10]

The bottom line is that God is the great Shepherd. God is inner healing. God is essential wholeness. God is a Father to the fatherless and a Defender of the widows. He will bring His justice against men who have misused and abused women. God will not bless you if you abuse your wife or other women because in so doing, is a contradiction to His nature.

Real men experience inner healing when they discover who God really is: an all-consuming Fire that heals the masculine soul, and not a dead, religious deity that can't handle the problems real men face on a daily basis. God is God.

In his book, *It's Not Over Until You Win!*, motivational speaker Les Brown states that "We all go through hard times. There have been periods in my life when my car was repossessed, the power to my house was shut off, and nobody believed in my dream. If I had accepted those times as permanent I would not be here now. There are times in life when it seems the harder you work, the deeper the hole you dig for yourself. But you've got to dig down deep within yourself and make a gut check. Whatever is pushing you down right now, you have to say I'm going to make it no matter what! [11]

4

WAKE UP, MEN

As Christian men, we must watch as well as pray, and be extremely careful with whom we align ourselves. We must not compromise the Christian faith, for there is only one Lord, one faith, and one baptism. Jesus Christ said, *"I am the way, the truth, and the life: no man cometh unto the Father, but by me"* (John 14:6).

I was a religion and philosophy major at Virginia Union University in Richmond, Virginia. I have a deep love for the great and diverse religions of the world. I firmly support the common link of monotheism, the belief in one God, which Christians, Jews, and Muslims share in the linkage to Abraham. Yet I bow and submit my life only to Jesus Christ because He is the one and only Savior, living Lord, and everlasting hope for the world.

On Christ the solid rock I stand, all other ground is sinking sand.

THE WINNING TEAM

A major source of inner healing for men is found in the fact that despite our daily setbacks and hardships as Christian men, we are still on the winning team. John 16:33 (Amplified): *"I have told you these things, so that in Me you may have (perfect) peace and confidence. In the world you have tribulations and trials and distress and frustration; but be of good cheer (take courage; be confident, certain, undaunted)! For I have overcome the world. (I have deprived it of power to harm you and have conquered it for you.)"*

I am so grateful to God that He speaks to me through His Word and gives my masculine soul inner healing and everlasting hope. Without words directly from the lips of God, my life would be worthless. For just one word from God empowers my spirit, soul, and body to press onward in the midst of the struggle and the good fight of faith. This struggle is a positive one, yet a painful one at times.

The true saint of God must be willing to lay his all on the line for the cause of Christ. The voice of God speaking directly to my heart heals the pain of rejection and personal persecution that persists. The Holy Spirit brings about an inner healing, a peace that passes all understanding, a quiet and blessed assurance in the midst of the storm.

In Christ Jesus I have this inner healing, inner peace, and peace of mind. Yes, the type of peace that passes all understanding. But in this world we will all have some troubles. Yes, I have personal trials and tribulations. So did Jesus, Moses, Joshua, Abraham, and Paul, as well as a host of other men with a mission and a God-ordained calling.

Trouble will certainly knock on the door of dedicated Christian men, especially when a man has surrendered his all to the Lord. It seems that troubles, trials, and tribulations decide to take up permanent residence in a man's life once he decides to get radically committed to Christ.

When a man gets serious about God's kingdom, Satan gets serious about slaying the man's spiritual lifestyle and relationship with the Lord. But don't worry; be happy. In fact, Jesus said, "Be of good cheer." Why? Because Jesus overcame this demonic world system full of its lies, hatred, lusts, greed, and illusions of boundless grandeur.

Christ, a Man above all men, the Savior of the world, gave His own life on an old, rugged cross of crucifixion and death. He rose again from the dead on the third day, conquering death, hell, and the grave.

So trials and tribulations will continue to come our way, but we have the victory because Jesus has defeated the devil, the author of all mass confusion. Stop the madness Satan has brought against your manhood, in the mighty name of Jesus. Tell the devil that you are taking back everything he stole from you.

It's time for men of destiny to take back their communities from dirty, old Beelzebub. It's time for us, as men of destiny, to take our streets and schools back from the clutches of Satan's control. It's time for us, as men of destiny, to take our children's souls back from the death grip of the fallen angel known as Lucifer. That type of positive action will provide a long overdue source of inner healing and essential wholeness for our communities, which are filled to the brim with inner turmoil and conflict.

WE ARE GOD'S CHILDREN

First John 4:4 (Amplified) says: *"Little children, you are of God (you belong to Him) and have (already) defeated and overcome them (the agents of the antichrist), because He Who lives in you is greater (mightier) than he who is in the world."*

It does not matter if you are a member of an Assemblies of God, Baptist, Catholic, Church of God in Christ, Episcopalian, Full Gospel, Independent, Lutheran, Methodist or Pentecostal denomination. If you are saved, washed in the blood of the Lamb, redeemed by the blood of Jesus, you're a child of God—even if you're a grown man.

It does not matter if you are a four-year-old boy, a forty-year-old man, or a 104-year-old senior gentleman. If you confess the Lord Jesus with your mouth, believe in your heart that He has risen from the dead, and repent of your sins, you are saved in the sight of almighty God. In God's eyes, the church, the chosen, the called-out ones, including the men, are His little children, and He is their Father.

As men, we must receive our inner healing and essential wholeness from the truth that because God is our heavenly Father and we are His children, then we are also natural-born overcomers. We can survive the storm, we can make it through the rough times, and we can overcome insurmountable obstacles, because the greater One, Jesus Christ, lives deeply within our hearts. We are not overcomers because of anything that we have done. We are overcomers who have found inner healing in the midst of hopelessness because the Spirit of Christ, the Overcomer of all hardships, lives in us. For in Him we live and move and have our being!

5

EFFECTIVE COMMUNICATION - INNER HEALING FOR MARRIED COUPLES

Effective communication is the key ingredient of develop-ing an atmosphere of inner healing for married men and women. Ineffective communication and insensitive spousal abuse cause millions of divorces. In fact, Scripture clearly speaks out against the evil treachery of spousal abuse. Malachi 2:14-16 de-clares, "Yet ye say, Wherefore? Because the Lord hath been witness between thee and the wife of thy youth, against whom thou hast dealt treacherously: yet is she thy companion, and the wife of thy covenant. And did not he make one? Yet had he the residue of the spirit. And wherefore one? That he might seek a godly seed. Therefore take heed to your spirit, and let none deal treacherously against the wife of his youth. For the Lord, the God of Israel, saith that he hateth putting away: for one covereth violence with his garment, saith the Lord of hosts: therefore take heed to your spirit, that ye deal not treacherously."

EFFECTIVE COMMUNICATION IS THE MAIN GOAL

Mere communication is not the objective in the ministry of inner healing and essential wholeness for married couples. Effec-tive communication is the main goal and objective in attaining inner healing in marriage. Empty and aimless chit-chat that contains no real, genuine concern for interpersonal relationships and totally lacks the true substance of sharing, caring, and nurturing for wounded married men and women is certainly the arch enemy of inner healing in marriage.

In the book, *I Have Heard From The Lord, And Sometimes God Sounds Like My Wife!*, Glenn Curtis Frazier Sr. gives an exceptional blueprint for inner healing in marriage:

"The institution of marriage rests on a relationship between two people, not one individual. Where there is only one person involved, there is no marriage. If only one person is responsible for all of the decisions, planning, labor, ideas, etc., then there is no need to get married. This kind of relationship is very frustrating to the other person who is not permitted to inject their ideas."[12]

Effective communication simply means that the message is received loud and clear with an understanding of what was said. If the message is not heard, is misunderstood, or is not explained clearly, it is not effective communication, which is the source of all inner healing.

For instance, the verbal and nonverbal communication skills of God, the spoken word and the actions of the Creator, are the ultimate source and motivating influence of inner healing in life. Because the Creator boldly declares that we are made in His image, we can overcome the negative verbal attacks and vicious labels people have placed on us in their utter ignorance of who we really are.

LISTENING AND RESPONDING AT THE RIGHT TIME

Effective communication requires the learned art of listening and responding at the right time and in the appropriate manner. In some cases, listening is all that is required to provide the needed release for a mate's inner healing. Other cases will absolutely require immediate action and consistent follow-up. The lack of effective communication is the death wish that wrenches the life out of marriages.

When couples learn to discuss issues and get a crystal clear understanding of putting into action the daily steps that it takes to make the marriage work, an atmosphere of inner healing for the marriage can slowly develop.

In his book, _Communication, Sex and Money_, Edwin Cole states: "The spirit in which we communicate seals all we say and do. God's love without Calvary would be so meaningless. A man's love without communication is so worthless. Be free to communicate. Cleanse your spirit with God's Word, and then release your spirit with your words. Confirm your words with gestures. Live your manhood to the fullest. Learn to communicate by word, gesture and spirit." [13]

Of course, the ultimate source of inner healing in marriage is realized in its fullest revelation through effective communication with God. Believers must spend daily quiet time alone in His presence. But we also need natural examples to grasp the more in-depth spiritual truths of inner healing for the wounded existence of married men and women in drastic need of meaning.

THE BASICS OF HOLISTIC MINISTRY TO YOUR SPOUSE

To make it plain and simple, you may love the Lord with all your heart, soul, and body, but don't fail to do some very basic things. Be concerned about the hurts of your spouse. Talk to and give gentle massages to them.

Maintain good personal hygiene on a daily basis, use deodorant, brush your teeth, keep that toilet seat clean, and dress neatly—even after the courtship is over. Husbands should also help out around the house, cooking and cleaning, and help with the children.

If we fail to deal with the basics of holistic ministry to our spouses when we have the power and opportunity to do so, our message of inner healing will be rendered useless because of a bad witness in the down-to-earth areas of life.

Men are motivated by sight, but women are mostly moved by touch and effective communication. The failure of a husband to effectively touch and communicate the message of inner healing, in word and deed, to his wife is the number one barrier and major roadblock to true intimacy in marriage. Remember that the man who causes his wife problems all day will have no peace at night.

Dr. Myles Monroe and David Burrows, in *Sex 101: Unlocking Hidden Truths about Sex,* say that sex and love are different. Sex is a desire (appetite). Love is a decision (commitment). They go on to say that "Love should be expressed sexually in the right time· and place; marriage."[14]

First Corinthians 7:3-6 states: *"Let the husband render unto the wife due benevolence: and likewise also the wife unto the husband. The wife hath not power of her own body, but the husband: and likewise also the husband hath not power of his own body, but the wife. Defraud ye not one the other, except it be with consent for a time, that ye may give yourselves to fasting and prayer; and come together again, that Satan tempt you not for your incontinence. But I speak this by permission, and not commandment."*

The walls that block all forms of effective verbal and nonverbal communication must be destroyed in order to develop the type of intimacy and anointed bonding that is ordained of God for marriage—the realization of being one flesh. Genesis 2:24 states, *"Therefore shall a man leave his father and his mother, and shall cleave unto his wife: and they shall be one flesh."*

REVIVAL IN THE HOME

"Flesh of my flesh and bone of my bones: I must discover oneness in marriage through effective communication. To become one flesh, I must overcome the selfish philosophy of only me, myself, and I."

Married couples must be unified through effective communication, prayer; working together and not against each other. Mark 10:6-9 states, _"But from the beginning of the creation God made them male and female. For this cause shall a man leave his father and mother, and cleave to his wife; And they twain shall be one flesh: so then they are no more twain, but one flesh. What therefore God hath joined together, let not man put asunder."_

Married couples need to work through the heated arguments and money matters, and use the most effective solutions, whether the man or the woman comes up with the right, God-ordained idea. As the head of the household, a husband also must give sight to the absolute truth that prayer, fasting, and effective communication with his wife are the only ways to achieve true and lasting inner healing in marriage.

A husband is called of God to keep revival going on in his home through effective communication with God, his wife, and his children. Author Steve Farrar says that when God changes a nation and brings revival, one of the primary things He does is to get a hold of some fathers and turn them into anchors.

In today's time of moral crises and fatherless America, Farrar writes, that's precisely what God is up to. God knows who His men are. He knows where they are and He knows who they are. He knows how to strongly support them. A husband is called to be the priest, provider, and protector for his wife and his children.

In other words, as the head of the household, the husband is called to be, above all, the servant of all. He should never negatively lord authority over his wife, but rather love her just as Christ loved the church and gave His very life for the church. That is true leadership in marriage. That means leadership in prayer in the home. That means leadership in fasting. That means leadership in family Bible study.

Farrar asks the thought-provoking question in **Anchor Man:** "How do you affect your family for the next one hundred years? By doing something today. By being obedient today. And then by doing something tomorrow. And one day those small deposits will begin to add up. Every time you love your wife as Christ loved the church, overtime you live with your wife in an understanding way, over time you grant your wife honor as fellow heir of the grace of life, you are putting away principal. It's like money in the bank." [15]

When a real man is willing to give of his own time and talent to be one flesh and love his wife as Christ loved the church, inner healing for married couples will realistically begin to occur in the land.

6

INNER HEALING FOR THE ABUSED

Considering the widespread forms of mental, verbal, and sexual abuse running rampant in countless families today, the subject of inner healing for the abused is extremely important and cannot be ignored.

When abuse first occurs the person is a victim, but if it is allowed to continue, the person becomes a volunteer for the continued abuse. God hates physical, mental, verbal, and sexual abuse. He wants to bring complete healing in the life of the family.

Abusers who are in denial must not be around their victims due to the harsh nature of their actions, especially in cases of physical and sexual abuse. It must be made very clear that every individual has the God-given right of free choice, whether right or wrong. God clearly calls on people to make the right choice, and there is a legal price and the price of God's anger to deal with when wrong choices are made concerning any form of abuse.

If there was physical, mental, verbal, or sexual abuse in your family, the best thing to do is break the cycle right now in the name of Jesus.

Many abusers have been abused themselves, but they can break the cycle. Just because someone's father beat the mother or children does not mean that the grown child of the abuser has to do the same. Get help. See a professional, Spirit-filled counselor.

The cycle of abuse can be destroyed in the name of Jesus, but the individual must first get inner healing. Then there can be inner healing for the family. For your own good, forgive the abuser for being so stupid to beat on another member of God's creation. Forgiving them is not saying that their abuse was right.

Rather, forgiving them is acknowledging that they totally ignored, did not fully realized, or just did not care at all that it is evil to abuse anybody. Forgiveness clears the path to the road of inner healing and essential wholeness. One does not have to agree with the wrong of abuser in order to forgive.

Jesus said of His tormentors: "Father, forgive them for they know not what they do." Anybody living in Jesus' day, with any common sense, would have known He was the wrong person to be messing around with, but Jesus used this moment to express the message of forgiveness.

There are many abusers who know exactly what they are doing. Therefore, every family member, even abusive family members, must accept Jesus as their own personal Lord and Savior. Anything else besides a personal relationship with Jesus that brings about accountability and personal conviction is a religious front and a pure waste of time.

God has only children—no grandchildren. We cannot get into heaven on our mother's, father's or grandparent's salvation. We must seek out our own soul salvation with fear and trembling. God wants to not only save each of us, but also our entire household.

Acts 16:31 states that *"And they said, Believe on the Lord Jesus Christ, and thou shalt be saved, and thy house."* God is clearly concerned about the family. There is no household that is not important to Him. Every single-parent home is at the top of God's priority list, every two-parent home is at the top of God's priority list, and every no-parent home is at the top of God's priority list.

Psalm 68:1 declares, *"Let God arise, let his enemies be scattered: let them also that hate him flee before him."* We must first let God arise in our lives individually before their can be any collective healing in the family of the church family. In other words: let God arise in your personal life, and let his enemies be scattered.

When Cain killed his brother, Abel, it was a classic case of not letting God arise, but letting hatred, bitterness, and anger arise. The arm of the flesh will never scattered the enemies of God. The healing power of God must arise first individually in the lives of family members in order to scatter personal demons and enemies of God that want to hold onto you for life.

Let God arise and let spousal abuse be scattered. Let God arise and let sexual abuse end. Let God arise, and let physical abuse end. Don't just talk about God, don't just sing about God and don't just preach about God. Instead, let God arise, and turn from the wicked ways of abusing the family.

No one should stay in an abusive relationship. The victim has the right to leave. When a person says no and you force yourself on them, that is rape. Let God arise and let His enemies of rape, spousal beatings, and verbal and mental torture be scattered. Not only must the victim forgive the abuser for their own soul survival, but it is the best way for them to go on with their own life.

The abuser also must ask for God's forgiveness, or else remain in the living hell of denial, and run the risk of passing on that satanic spirit of family abuse to someone else. The key word for the abuser is repent. You might be in jail for the rest of your life, but still repent and at least you will have the promise of eternal life with Jesus Christ. Abuser, you may have lost your family, but you don't have to lose your soul. Living in denial only furthers the torture of your soul.

Let God arise and let His enemies that ruined all your relationships be scattered. In today's world, no one, nobody, has to sit
around and be abused. The victim is not required by God at all to
take that mess.

To folks who were abused in their past: don't bring abuse into
your own family and your future. Learn to discipline with firm love.
Learn effective, loving ways to discipline your child. You can find
many good parenting books at the library or a Christian bookstore,
maybe even your church's library.

Different forms of discipline include distracting a toddler or
preschooler to something else; putting a youngster in time-out for
a few minutes; withdrawing a privilege from an older child, such as
going out to play; or, giving a child a restrained, controlled spank-
ing on the bottom. Some parenting experts recommend that if you
choose to spank, use just one or two swats on the bottom—not
with your hand—but with an inanimate object such as a wooden
spoon from the kitchen. Whichever form of discipline you use,
always conclude the episode with verbally reaffirming to your child
your unconditional love for them. Never hit in a fit of anger.

Let your past abuse be in the past, let it stop now, and not be
passed onto another generation. Physical, sexual, mental, and verbal abuse is an expression of hatred toward all that God represents.
Let those actions that display hatred toward the ways of God flee
from His presence. It cannot be pushed under the rug. Physical,
mental, verbal, and sexual abuse are a reality.

The family is also in drastic need of inner healing and essential
wholeness, and the Bible clearly points out how it can be received.
Psalms 68:5 states that "A father of the fatherless, and a judge of the
widows, is God in his holy habitation."

Our body is the temple of God and our praises unto Him is also
His holy habitation. God inhabits the praises of His people. God
will be a Father to the fatherless and a Defender to the widow. God
can fill the void in our life that no one else can, because He is God. ·

Youngsters who don't have a father in their home are more likely to get in trouble with the law. But, God said He will be a Father to the fatherless. God says, "I have not forgotten about that daughter or son without a dad. They're going to make it. They will succeed. They will survive. I will be the Father they never had. I will never give up on any of My children."

As well as remembering the fatherless son and daughter, God remembers the forgotten widow. He promises to bring justice to her situation. God is concerned about inner healing for men and women because He wants to heal the entire family.

Psalm 68:6 gives us some keys points concerning inner healing for the family: "*God setteth the solitary in families: he bringeth out those which are bound with: but the rebellious dwell in a dry land.*" God puts, He places, He literally sets the solitary people—meaning the lonely, as in locked-down in solitary confinement—in families.

God planned for you to be in the family that you are in. He set the solitary, the lonely, in families where they could get the most help. Some people get the most help from their blood family. Others get more help from their church family, or close friends, but God always sets the lonely in families where there is someone who can let them know that they are lonely but not alone.

It may be a grandmother, a father, a brother, a pastor, or a sister of brother in Christ, but there will always be someone God uses to show His love to you, and give you a true sense of family. No matter how lonely you are, God has you in that family for a reason. He wants to heal you and your family. He wants to heal you and your entire household. The same blood of Jesus that saves from the deepest sin also heals the deepest wounds within the spirit, soul, and body. Healing has come to your house.

Scripture says that "he bringeth out those which are bound with chains." Get ready to come out of the solitary confinement of the wounded spirit and soul. Grab hold of God's hand because He is going to bring you out. Make a financial budget because God is

47

going to bring you out. Pay off all your smallest bills first because God is going to bring you out. Get your priorities straight because God is going to bring you out.

God is going to bring you out of debt, out of bad relationships, out of promiscuity, out of homosexuality, out of lesbianism, out of adultery, out of fornication. God brings out those who are bound with chains. You have been bound to sin too long.

Praise God! He will take the shackles off your feet so you can dance. He will remove the chains of drugs, alcohol, lying, cheating, and stealing. Be loosed, be set free in the mighty name of Jesus. Praise God from whom all blessings flows for your deliverance. Praise Him for your breakthrough.

The rebellious dwell in a dry land. The family member who is lonely, and locked down in the solitary confinement of their soul, but seeks the face of God will be released by the Master. They will decide not to rebel against the God who delivered them.

This is something to rejoice in because there are many family members who will rebel against God. Scripture says the rebellious will dwell in a dry land. They will have to live with themselves and their rebellion against God who wanted to heal them.

You can be healed only if you receive healing; only if you want it. God will never force it on you. If you want to stay angry, and blame everyone else except yourself, you will never receive healing. Healing comes by realizing that only God can bring about true inner healing and essential wholeness. In some cases you have to wipe the dust off your feet and leave people in the hands of God.

7

INNER HEALING THROUGH THE MOVE OF GOD

J oel 2:28 says, *"And it shall come to pass afterward, that I will pour out My Spirit upon all flesh; and your sons and daughters shall prophesy, your old men shall dream dreams, and your young men shall see visions; and also upon the servants and upon the handmaids in those days will I pour out My Spirit."*

We need to allow the Holy Spirit to move into our lives and take up permanent residency within our human spirit. Otherwise other things will take up residency: hatred, animosity, jealousy, and all different types of demons.

The Bible says that once a demon is cast out of a person, if they don't live right, that same demon can return; only this time it will come back with seven more demons and they will form a satanic stronghold within that individual.

As men in need of meaning, we need God's delivering power. There are things occurring within each and every one of our lives that we know that are not right with God. He wants us to yield our lives to Him. So many people say, "Preacher, what does it mean to yield my life to God?"

Well, it's like getting on a boat, in a stream or an ocean, and not paddling yourself, but going with the flow of the stream. That's what it's like to yield to God. We don't like doing it because, as men, we like to be in control. We like things to go exactly according to plan.

Even in church, we want the Sunday service to go exactly by the program. God does not work that way! We cannot limit Him to a program, we cannot limit Him to what we have put down in writing. His Holy Spirit wants to move in people's lives, because He's aware of the problems and the predicaments and the challenges going on.

In the Christian classic, *How to Bring Men to Christ*, R. A. Torrey shares the insight that, "Obedience means more than the mere performance of some of the things God commands us to do. It means the entire surrender of our wills, ourselves, and everything we have to Him."[16]

It's the moving of the Holy Spirit in our lives individually and collectively as men of destiny that births inner healing in our wounded souls. We need to be concerned, not just about our personal destiny and success, with what God is doing corporately in the church body. God moves in your life and bless you individually so you can be a blessing to somebody else.

He doesn't want us to keep that blessing to ourselves. We may have some conference tapes or a few books, or maybe there are some Scriptures that God has revealed to you in a new way. Your spirit has been touched. As men of God, He wants us to share those things with somebody else.

Jesus wants us to spread that fire. He doesn't want us to keep that fire (that move of God) to ourselves. He wants us to share it so it can touch somebody else's life. God is a God that moves within people. He just doesn't move in your life individually and leaves it up to only you. He moves in the lives of His people. He didn't touch and speak to Joel and then never had Joel share that message with anyone else.

God dealt with Joel and then God dealt with Joel to write what He told him to write so it could touch other people's lives down through the ages. God is not a selfish God. He never wants us to keep all the Word, all the blessings to ourselves.

YIELD CONTROL TO GOD

There is a human condition that all of us have gone through at one time or another: hopelessness. Our back is up against the wall and we cannot turn the situation around ourselves. That's the time God wants us to yield to Him. That's the time He wants us to get on that "boat" of trust and faith and let Him control our lives.

Many people don't want to lift up their hands and praise God because if they can just hold down their hands and move them the way they want to, they're in control. However, lifting up your hands is a sign of yielding to God. Lifting up your hands is an outward, physical sign of yielding—totally surrendering—your life to God.

Many men have been abused and molested and have so many negative things troubling their spirit. They feel they cannot re-lease the deep pain and fear to God. But, my brother, God wants you to release the control to Him.

When we talk about God being in control, is He really in con-trol in our lives—in every area? Is God really moving in your life? Have you found true inner healing or is it just a show, a form of godliness that denies the power thereof?

You probably got up this morning and put on your work clothes or business suit, your work shoes or dress shoes. You maybe even helped get the children fed and dressed. Then you got in the car and headed for work or maybe church. Was it all in vain?

It was—and is—in vain if we don't allow God to prevail and have the preeminence in our lives. It's all in vain if we don't allow Him to be the Lord of our life—the Lord of our tongues, the Lord of our eyes, the Lord of our hands, the Lord of our actions.

We have to get to that point where God takes full control of our lives. Where we say that our doctrine is for Him. Many folks don't want to give on that stuff, yet a holy God will begin to deal with those things in our life that we know are not right. We wonder why we don't receive the blessings of God. Well, what's going on in our lives? Let's take a long, hard look—individually and collectively—and maybe we'll find out the exact reasons why God cannot bless us.

MEN OF DESTINY

God could not bless the children of Israel because of the sin of one. Until Joshua dealt with the sins in the camp, God could not bless His people. Even today, one person can be lying, one person can be sleeping around, one person can be gossiping on the phone, and God will not bless.

You may think that's not right, that it's not biblical. But it's in this context that God begins to deal with Joel about the sins of the children of Israel. In Joel 1:8 it says, *"Lament like a virgin girded with sackcloth for the husband of her youth,"* meaning longing.

We must long for the move of God, like a virgin that longs for a relationship with the husband of her youth, by keeping herself pure. She waits for the ecstasy and the blessing, not only in a sexual sense, but also in a sense of knowing the person in every aspect that they can be known.

How much time do we spend talking with the Lord? How much time do we spent in His presence? We say that we know the Lord, but the Bible says there will be many who say, "Lord, I prophesied in your Name, I preached in your Name, I cast out demons in your Name." God's response will be for them to depart because He doesn't know them.

You can tell a lot about a person's relationship with God and the depth of it by their conversation. You'll know a tree by the fruit that it bears. If you're getting into the things of God, there are certain things your conscience or your spirit will convict you of.

You may still think certain things, you may still want to do certain things, but you'll be convicted by the Holy Spirit not to say or do them. This is what happens when God's Holy Spirit is moving upon the waters of your human spirit.

Has Jesus been knocking on the doors of your heart and you refuse to let Him in? Beware, you may have instead let in that demon. The difference can be told through your tongue. The Bible says, "Out of the abundance of the heart the mouth speaks." From our conversation people can tell what's going on spiritually in our life.

The passage from Joel continues: "Lament like a virgin girded with sackcloth for the husband of her youth; the meat offering and the drink offering is cut off from the house of the Lord; the priests, the Lord's ministers, mourn. The field is wasted, the land mourneth; for the corn is wasted; the new wine of the Holy Spirit, is dried up, the oil languisheth. Be ye ashamed, oh ye husbandmen; howl. The creature howls.

"Oh ye vinedressers, the church, for the wheat and for the barley; because the harvest of the field is perished. The soul that once was saved, that's where. The field, the wheat, the barley has perished.

But God is saying that I want to move by My Spirit. He says, "The vine is dried up, and the fig tree languisheth; the pomegranate tree, the palm tree also, and the apple tree, even all the trees of the field are withered; because the joy is withered away from the sons of men."

We must not let anybody steal our joy. This joy that I have, the world didn't give it to me, the world didn't give it, and the world can't take it away. So we've got to understand that the joy of the Lord is our strength.

SACRIFICES OF PRAISE

When we start praising God, we make His heart joyful and in turn He gives us strength and inner healing to make it through the day and any frustrations. As men we're trying to do it ourselves, but God is saying, "I want to move through you. I want you to totally yield yourself to Me."

We normally just don't do that in the natural, but this is an example in the spiritual where what we need, God can do. That is, if we really want God to be in control.

Joel says, "Gird yourselves, and lament, ye priests." God wants ministers to intercede, to cry out to God because of the conditions going on in the world and in our own community. "Ye ministers of. my God; for meat offering and the drink offering is withholden from the house of your God."

In Joel's time they offered up to God sacrifices of meat—lambs, bulls, etc. We don't have to do that today. Romans 14:17 says, "*For the kingdom of God is not meat and drink, but righteousness and peace and joy in the Holy Ghost.*" We need to understand what's going on in our lives as men and what Scripture is saying. We don't have to offer up sacrifices of meat anymore because Jesus became the ultimate sacrifice on Calvary. However, we ought to give Him our sacrifices of praise! We ought to give Him the fruit of our heart!

In Joel 2:1, it says, "*Blow ye the trumpet in Zion, and sound the alarm in My holy mountain; let all the inhabitants of the land tremble; for the day of the Lord cometh, for it is nigh at hand.*"

THE TIME OF OUR VISITATION AND THE VALLEY OF DECISION

In understanding the move of God, we must understand that if we don't yield ourselves as men to God and a visitation of His Holy Spirit, we miss out. We miss our time of visitation and we also have to then face the judgment of God.

On one hand, there's the move of God: a major Source of true inner healing; all that God is trying to do in our lifetime; and, His many abundant blessings. On the other hand, there's the judgment of God. The Bible says that "it's appointed unto man once to die, and then the judgment."

In the book of Joel, the judgment of God is called "the day of the Lord." Joel 3:14 says, *"Multitudes, multitudes in the valley of decision,"* the day of the Lord is near in the valley of decision. The valley of decision is the valley of Jehoshaphat, it is the valley of judgment.

This isn't the decision we make ourselves. This is the decision God makes. This same valley of decision in Joel is alluded to in Revelation. Revelation 4:1 says, *"a door is opened in heaven,"* and it says that God is sitting upon the throne. There are the twenty-four elders with Him and the seven Spirits of God, or personalities of God.

Twelve of the twenty-four represent the patriarchs of the Old Testament. Twelve represents the apostles of the New Testament. God is the judge sitting on the throne and the jury is the twelve from the Old, and the twelve from the New. But this thing is real.

Some folks say, "All my life I've been hearing that Jesus is coming back and He hasn't come back yet." That's the most foolish statement anybody could make. They don't understand that "to be absent from the body is to present with the Lord." Once somebody who is a true believer dies, they're in Christ, they're with the Lord. When a non-believer dies, they go before the great throne of judgment. It happens instantaneously. So to us, hundreds of years may have gone by, but to them they are instantly there in the seat of judgment.

This thing is real. As men of destiny we have to listen to what God is saying. Continuing in Joel, it says, "Blow the trumpet in Zion, sanctify a fast, and call a solemn assembly." Sometimes we have to put down our plates and begin to fast, and say, "God, I want you to move in my life. I know there are some things that are not right. I don't like the direction I'm going in."

My brother, you will be led by somebody, whether you like it or not. Somebody will be in control of your life, whether or not you're fully aware of it. If you don't yield yourself to the move of God,

Satan will send somebody to influence you in such a negative way that you'll find yourselves doing things you never said you would do.

HIS SPIRIT ON ALL FLESH

I'm here to tell you that there must be some maintenance. Watch with whom you spend your time. If you're always around somebody who is talking about God, pretty soon you'll be talking about God. It's one thing to try and witness to non-believers, if you are strong in the Lord. But if you are trying to spend all your time with them and you're being fed their negative conversation, pretty soon you're going to be pulled down in the gutter, too. As the saying goes: "If you sleep with dogs, you'll turn up with fleas."

Verse 28 says, *"And it shall come to pass afterwards, I will pour out My Spirit upon all flesh."* After you have yielded yourself to the Lord; after you have submitted yourself, it says He will pour out His Spirit on all flesh.

It doesn't say He will pour out His Spirit on only black people; it says, "all flesh." If we have a service and invite somebody to speak, maybe to preach to those white people, don't stay home. God said He was going to pour out His Spirit on all flesh.

No matter what color anybody is, if they're preaching God's Word. They could have could something that can be a blessing to your life. "Receive ye the Word of the Lord."

Joel says the Spirit of God will move on all flesh; that "your sons and daughters shall prophesy." So, my brother, here the Bible is dealing with sexism. It doesn't say that just your boys are going to prophesy, it says your daughters will, too.

Some people say that's the only passage in the entire Bible that includes women doing ministry. However, throughout the Old and New Testament there are many instances of women going forth to do the work of God. We have to deal with the sexism.

In addition, other folks, out of ignorance, say that Christianity is the white man's religion. Again, that's the farthest thing from the truth. The Bible is the only spiritual book that has the presence of the black man in it and gives respect to women. You don't find any other spiritual books that have names of women within them, the Bible has two: Esther and Ruth. The Bible deals with the racism and it deals with the sexism, it deals with it all. We don't have to run to anybody to get the answer. God gives us the answer in His Word, the holy Bible.

DREAM AND VISIONS

If we run to God's Word, He will give us the answer. Joel 2 says, *"Your sons and daughters,"* then it says, *"your old men shall dream dreams and your young men shall see visions."* Younger men should not intimidate older men. We have to understand the times and the seasons of our life. There is a time when God wants us—a young person up to about the age of twenty-five—to learn all we can. Get as much education as you can, gather all the information you can.

Don't run off and get with this girlfriend or boyfriend. Have some friends, but get all the knowledge that you can. Prepare yourself. Then, when you're about twenty-five years of age, find and work at your career, your vocation in life. Sometime in there settle down, get married and have a family. Go forth and do your life's work—what God has called you to do. Be a blessing to others.

Then, in the later years of life, such as around fifty, and as you head toward retirement age, share with young men all that you've learned in life. Plant seeds in others. Help them to discover the purpose that God has for them.

Joel says, "Old men will dream dreams." Dreams might be fulfilled, but dreams are not promised to be fulfilled. It also says, "Young men shall see visions." If the Bible says it, it means it. If it says you will see visions, it means you will see visions come to pass, even if you have to wait until you are ninety-nine years old. However, I don't think this passage really deals with chronological age as much as the spiritual seasons in a person's life.

Men, learn to pray this prayer: "Holy Spirit, breathe on me. Holy Spirit, breathe in me. Holy Spirit, breathe through me for You are my Source of inner healing."

8

THE STRENGTH OF SMALL BEGINNINGS

Today's church, the entire corporate body of Christ, severely needs a precise course of action that will lead to a higher level of success through struggle. Remember that struggle, perseverance, and determination are all mandatory steps toward fulfilling your personal, your spiritual destiny.

In the Book of Acts, throngs of people where daily added to the church. The apostles wrought tremendous exploits through the power of God because the early church understood their destiny. The early church also had a plan of action directly based upon their call to destiny.

Their course of action was to preach in the power of the name of Jesus, and to yield their lives to God through the power of the Holy Spirit. The early church was on its mission to reach the masses with the gospel of Jesus Christ.

Today, these methods may seem old, out of date, and antiquated, but they are not. The same God who reigned in the days of the apostles still sits on the throne today. Hebrews 13:8 says, *"Jesus Christ the same yesterday, today, and forever more."*

Despite all the seminars, conventions, crusades, and revivals we have available to us today, it cannot compare to the Holy Ghost power that flowed through the early church. However, today's church still has the same mandate and destiny to win the world for Christ. As men of God how can we accomplish such a goal? How can today's church make an impact for Christ amid our fast-paced, high-tech, and crises-laden society?

FOLLOW THE FOOTSTEPS OF JESUS

First of all, we need to follow in the footsteps of Jesus. Jesus ministered a message of inner healing and essential wholeness to people at their level. The church also must come down to earth in order to reach everyday ordinary people. Christ developed His ministry by constantly investing into the lives of the twelve disciples.

Jesus walked with twelve men in need of a Messiah. Jesus talked with these men. Jesus ate with them. Jesus motivated them as no other man could. He used the twelve disciples to help Him fulfill His destiny that ultimately led to the old rugged cross at Calvary. These twelve ordinary men did not fully understand their Friend's divine calling until they became apostles, after the resurrection.

Yet Jesus daily poured His heavenly philosophy for victorious living in real life situations into their spirits. Through this divine concept of investing in the lives of the disciples, Jesus reached hundreds of thousands of men, women, boys, and girls for the kingdom of God. Jesus wan not sexist and we must not be sexist either.

In his book, *Brothers! Calling Men into Vital Relationships*, Geoff Gorsuch states: "The process of building vital relationships among men can be likened to a baseball diamond in that there are four phases of development. The process starts as we step up to the plate with the desire and the determination to become more like Christ. Then the men become acquainted with each other at first base. At second base, the relationships progress to the level of friendship. From there, we round third base and head toward home plate as communication and commitment to one another deepen. Thus, we become the brothers Christ intends us to be."[17]

In fact when Jesus Christ began His church, He multiplied the number of disciples by ten, and formally gave His stamp of approval on the beginnings of the church through the baptism of the Holy Spirit when there were one hundred and twenty in one accord. The Holy Spirit will move miraculously through inner healing in the midst of the church when the body of Christ is in one accord.

The course of action the church must take is to be like Jesus and to personally invest in small groups—such as the twelve disciples or the one hundred and twenty in the upper room—and thereby develop a support system to effectively reach the masses for God's kingdom. Jesus had a pretty good track record: He had only one person in His nucleus group who turned on Him. Turnover is a major concern, but if you're investing in men's small groups through the guidance of the Holy Spirit, God will open doorways of destiny. He'll lead you to reach others through the personalities and gifts of the members of your small group.

Small Beginnings Builds Great Substance

When you look at any major church, ministry, or business, most of the successful ones did not start off that way. Most of them started with a small nucleus of people, men and women of destiny, who invested biblical principles of success within their people. This motivated them to greatness within their given organization.

The direction today's church must go in, to make a lasting impact on our culture, is to clearly remember not to despise the day of small beginnings. Small beginnings are the foundation needed to fulfill destiny and God's message of inner healing. Even people who don't come from small beginnings need to acquire the experience to develop compassion in ministering to the hurting and the wounded.

Small beginnings actually build the substance and character needed to develop major movements that make a difference in a spiritually starving world. In other words major movements of destiny that reach the masses are birthed and nurtured through the influence of small groups whose philosophy for living raises the consciousness of the people.

In order for this to work, the church must first excel in the truth and integrity of God's Word. Many church leaders don't get even near the doorway of their destiny because they don't believe the major teachings of the Bible. Any church that does not believe in the truth and integrity of God's Word is not a true New Testament Church and will not fulfill their God-given destiny. The only church that has a future of succeeding in the kingdom of God is the church that is led by the wounded Savior. We need churches to relate and reach out to wounded people with every day, real life problems. Any church that ignores this reality will die. Any church that consistently addresses these issues through the leading of the Holy Spirit, will prosper.

Rejoice in the day of small beginnings. Pray fervently for all pastors, teachers, prophets, apostles, and evangelists—both male and female. Support them fully in the work of the ministry.

Our church programs must offer a way to get the wounded through the door. We cannot leave them outside, bleeding and vulnerable to the evil beast of society who wants to steal their joy and rob them of their inner healing. We must reach out to the old and young backslider saints who still have seeds of destiny within them. Let's encourage and compel them concerning their part in God's overall program.

Whoever comes through your church doors, invest God's Word in them—the Word that never returns void. Mentor them. Disciple them. Nurture them. Love them, and even when you think all hope is gone, God will open doors.

Men, learn to rejoice in the day of small beginnings. Jesus started His mission with only twelve ordinary men. Down through the ages to today, it has reached and touched countless millions of lives.

9

Keep On Climbing My Brother

Genesis 28 contains a well-known story concerning a strange dream Jacob, the son of Isaac, had one night. In the dream Jacob saw a ladder set up on the earth with the top of the ladder reaching up to the very portal of glory in heaven. Jacob saw angels descending and ascending on that trusty ladder. (Gen. 28:12).

God, the Father of life and hope, outlined Jacob's divinely ordained, strategized destiny to him through this very unique dream. Genesis 28:13-15 describes in detail what God said to Jacob:

13 *"And behold, the Lord stood above it, and said, I am the Lord God of Abraham thy father, and the God of Isaac; the land whereon thou liest, to thee will I give it, and to thy seed;*

14 *And thy seed shall be as the dust of the earth, and thou shalt spread abroad to the west, and to the east, and to the north, and to the south: and in thee and in thy seed shall all the families of the earth be blessed.*

15 *And, behold, I am with thee in all places whither thou goest, and will bring thee again into this land; for I will not leave thee, until I have done that which I have spoken to thee of."*

That is a classic example of divine destiny established by the Creator, to be executed by His children. That is a message with deep implications of inner healing and essential wholeness for the tortured and troubled masculine soul. God put a seed of destiny in Jacob's loins and told him, in essence, "I won't leave you alone, until My will and My Word to you is accomplished."

We cannot run or hide from the predestined plan and purpose of God. When it is all said and done, He will have all eminence, praise, and glory due His holy name.

Let's remember that Jacob was the dirty old liar who stole his brother, Esau's, birthright just a chapter ago at the recommendation of his deceitful dear mother, Rebekah. Jacob ended up paying a dear price for his crime: his brother hated him for life, and became the source and seed that provided the birth of many of Israel's most notorious enemies.

Also, Jacob never again saw his mother. She died outside of the camp of God's perfected will and plan.

A Peculiar Dream Reveals God's Perfect Plan

Even though Jacob knew this peculiar dream represented God's perfect, predestined plan, he still was required to get off his rear end and do some work in order to fulfill God's plan. He had to grab hold of this dream concerning a ladder that led to a far greater destination than this old world. How do you think divine destiny is realized? By osmosis? No, it's by rolling up our sleeves and taking care of business. That is why God told Jacob, "I will not leave thee, until I have done that which I have spoken to thee of." God was going to do it through Jacob, an ordinary man. Jacob was the vessel of destiny even though his empty vessel was broken, battered, and bruised. God uses ordinary men for extraordinary purposes to enhance and promote the causes of the kingdom.

When Jacob woke up, he immediately said, in dreadful terror of the awesome revelation from God, that *"this is none other but the house of God, and this is the gate of heaven"* (Gen. 28:17). In other words, the revelation was of angels ascending and descending on a ladder leading to the house of God—directly to the gates of heaven, a divine doorway of destiny.

When the American slaves, the seeds of the motherland Africa, struggled under the whip of oppression, brutality, and blatant injustice, they would bravely sing "We are climbing Jacob's ladder, we are climbing Jacob's ladder, we are climbing Jacob's ladder, soldiers of the cross." As they sang that song they most definitely had a greater destiny in view.

True Revival that Brings Deep Inner Healing

My beloved brothers of divine destiny, each day they struggled for the cause of Christ, and walked by faith in an unseen God, they were somehow one day closer to destiny, and freedom from the brutal and vicious bondage of being enslaved in American.

Yet, there is a new slavery in America. All of our major political, religious, and community leaders have addressed and discussed it, but still nothing has really changed because they don't have the power to appropriate the inner healing balm, and fresh oil of God. Government cannot eradicate the degrading behavioral pattern that has its deep roots in the sins of the past—images promoted by years of slavery, bigotry, and racial hatred.

Blaming the white man is not the solution. True revival that brings deep inner healing to the wounded masculine heart and soul and literally changes the hearts, minds and very core nature of the races is the only solution to our present day predicament concerning the fury of racial wars and conflict.

Today, the same God of Abraham, Isaac, Jacob, Charles Finney, Smith Wigglesworth, Kathryn Kuhlman, Sojourner Truth, Frederick Douglas and Dr. Martin Luther King Jr., is calling on today's entire

Christian church body to hold on and take a climb, climbing up Jacob's ladder. This is a ladder that leads to heaven's door.

10

STANDING IN THE GAP

Ezekiel 22: 23-31: "*And the word of the Lord came unto me, saying, Son of man, say unto her, Thou art the land that is not cleansed, nor rained upon in the day of indignation. There is a conspiracy of her prophets in the midst thereof, like a roaring lion ravening the prey; they have devoured souls; and they have taken the treasure and precious things, they have made her many widows in the midst thereof. Her priests have violated my law, and have profaned mine holy things: they have put no difference between the holy and profane, neither have they shewed difference between the unclean and the clean, and have hid their eyes from my Sabbaths, and I am profaned among them. "Her princes in the midst thereof are like wolves ravening the prey, to shed blood, and to destroy souls, to get dishonest gain. And her prophets have daubed them with untempered mortar, seeing vanity, and deviling lies unto them, saying, Thus saith the Lord God, when the Lord hath not spoken. The people of the land have used oppression, and exercised robbery, and have vexed the poor and needy: yea, they hive oppressed the stranger wrongfully. And I sought for a man among them, that should make up the hedge, and stand in the gap before me for the land, that I should not destroy it; but I found none. Therefore have I poured out mine indignation upon them; I have consumed them with the fire of my wrath; their own way have I recompensed upon their heads, saith the Lord God."*

This passage of Scripture deals with God's judgment on the children of Israel.

From the pulpit to the door and beyond, the Creator was unpleased with His children, with His creation. In essence, God said, there is a conspiracy in the midst of His people. A conspiracy is a plan to connive; to not focus on the name of the Lord, but to lift up personalities and attitudes. Even today, we see this as a reality. Scripture lets us know that the judgment begins in the household of God.

In *Courage: A Book for Champions*, Edwin Cole writes, "Men who know how to pray exercise a boldness toward life that enables them to be more that conquerors. They know God is for them, they need not fear anyone who is against them." Dr. Cole also says, "The result of prayer in private will be a life of boldness and courage in public."[18]

THE HOLY AND THE PROFANE

It behooves us to listen to the words of the Scripture writer, to find out what the Lord wants to speak to the church concerning His destiny, plan and purpose for each and every one of our personal lives. Scripture talks of a time in which the law of the Lord is being violated. He uses these words, that they "have profaned, have cursed Holy things, and there is no difference in between the Holy and the profane."

There is a difference between being in the center of God's will and straddling the fence. As people of God, we must lift up our voices and love everyone. But even in loving them, even in showing forth the mercy of God, we must take a stand as blood brought believers.

We have a cotillion at our church where the young women share various poems, songs, and other things they have learned in

Young Women's Fellowship. Our young men share things they have learned in Young Men's Fellowship. But over in Bosnia, Herzegovina, they had a beauty pageant and asked the winner, "What do you want to do since you have won this crown?" Her response: "I'm not concerned what I'm going to do because I don't even know if I'll be alive tomorrow."

GOD IS SEARCHING FOR A MAN

In the midst of all the turmoil that is going on in the world, God is searching for a man— single or married—that lives in the midst of the turmoil and the frustration of the moment.

God is saying, "I have searched to and fro, throughout the earth, looking to find a man." Many people would say this is speaking in the generic sense that it is speaking of men who would answer the call of the Lord. That is true, but in our society and in our situation, we must emphasize that God is searching for a man who will stand up for truth.

Thank God for all the men who are faithful to the cause of Christ. But the Lord needs even more men to stand up and fulfill their divine destiny. God is searching for a man who will stand up among them.

My brothers of purpose, this is the reason for the entire church: to build up a wall of righteousness in the world today. There clearly is a wall of unrighteousness, but the Lord wants to raise up a standard against the works of Satan.

To save the youth of today, we must stand up and be the men of God that the Lord has called us to be. The Lord has called for us to fulfill our plan and purpose of destiny in God in order for the youth to be who they should be, and for women to be whom they should be.

I know it's tight, but it's totally right. The Lord is searching out for men of destiny to take their place, proclaim a word of inner healing to broken marriages, homes and families to take their position in God. I said it many times, we all have ministry. My ministry may not be like yours, your ministry may not be like mine, but we must find our place, our predestined plan, and our purpose in God.

Revelation 3:8 says *"I know thy works: behold, I have set before thee an open door, and no man can shut it."* God wants men to walk through the doorway of destiny and fill up the vacancy, fill up the empty spaces, and fill up the hedges and gaps in our community, and in our homes, for our children are dying. There are too many young people already planning their funerals and not their God-given destiny. The Lord needs a man to stand up and to stand firm.

CALLING ALL INTERCESSORS

My Brother, this is about intercession; this is about inner healing for the wounded masculine soul. Intercession means you are interceding on behalf of someone else who cannot help themselves in their situation. It means you are "standing in" for them. It means you are standing in proxy for them because they're in a tough situation in which there's no way out; their back is up against the wall.

More specifically, it means you're standing in proxy for a drug addict, a liar, a thief, a backslidden church member, a prisoner, a homeless person.

One of the first prophets on the scene, Isaiah, also bore witness to what Ezekiel said. In Isaiah 59:16, Isaiah said, *"And he saw that there was no man, and wondered that there was no intercessor:"* The Lord wants ordinary men to intercede, the Lord wants men to "stand in the gap," for that male prostitute standing on the corner. The Lord wants men to "stand in the gap" for that son or daughter who robbed the liquor store. The Lord wants men to "stand in the gap" for that young man holding a forty-ounce bottle of malt liquor. The Lord wants men to "stand in the gap." Somebody might say, "How can I stand in the gap, Rev. Mackey?"

THE SPIRIT HELPS OUR INFIRMITIES

Romans 8:26 says, *"Likewise the Spirit also helpeth our infirmities: for we know not what we should pray for as we ought: but the Spirit itself maketh intercession for us with groanings which cannot be uttered. So we will not always know what to pray for."*

Sometimes we're down on our knees, interceding, and we're actually angry at the person we're standing in for because they're messing up so badly. Our prayers may be judgmental, but God does not want us to judge any man, only ourselves. We need to keep our own house in order. When we get into this realm of the Spirit, realizing that Jesus sent the Holy Spirit to be a Comforter, then we can realize that the Spirit also helps our infirmities.

Jesus knows all about our troubles. The Spirit knows the situation and what our loved ones are going through. The Spirit understands things that have gone on for many years and how that have affected people's psyche. The Spirit of God will teach us to make intercession so that God can also open doors in their lives. The Spirit of God will teach us to stand in the gap, through groanings that cannot be uttered. Sometimes when we have to go down into the gap, it is like going down into the sewer because the situation gets dirty.

But, the Spirit of Jesus will help us walk through the water. There may be things that prevent us from going on, but the Spirit will lead the way. We have to get down on our knees and call on the name of Jesus. Sometimes we won't know what or how to pray. So, we simply groan and rock from side to side. We pray. "I don't know how You're going to work it out, Lord, but I give it over to You."

Are you willing to stand in the gap so Jesus can open doorways of destiny for the deprived, despised, disenfranchised, and disinherited members of society? Jesus Christ cared about the outcast. Why don't we? Many of the men in the jail and on the street corner, they could be our future doctors, lawyers, physicians, architects, but somebody has to stand in the gap for them.

Somebody has to build up a wall of righteousness by getting down on their knees and interceding with some powerful prayer. Somebody has to burn some midnight oil and call out to the name of the Lord.

The name of Jesus has power. It has influence, clout, and credibility beyond compare. The name of Jesus opens doors that no one else can ever close! Romans 27:8 says, *"And he that searcheth the hearts knoweth what is the mind of the Spirit, because he maketh intercession for the saints according to the will of God."*

Get caught up with the Comforter in the name of Jesus Christ. It's the Holy Spirit that teaches the saints to make intercession in the will of God. Feel the Spirit of the Lord move in your life. Become an intercessor. Become a last day warrior. Put on the helmet of salvation, put on the breastplate of righteousness, have your feet shod with the preparation of the gospel of peace, and hold up high the sword of the Spirit.

A BATTLE IS GOING ON

A battle is going on, but the battle is not ours, but it is the Lord's. Be prepared to wait on Him. We have to learn to call on Him. We have to learn to cry out to Him in intercessory prayer. God will hear us as we come to the foot of the cross and He will answer. God is calling us to stand in the gap today. God is calling us to say, "Here I am, Lord, send me. I'm willing to go. I'm willing to endure hardship. I'm willing to endure criticism. Lord, I'm willing to do Your will. Yes, Lord!" If we do not stand in the gap, we will suffer the consequences greatly. Listen to the voice of prophecy in God's Word: "And I sought for a man among them, that should make up the hedge, and stand in the gap before me for the land, and I should not destroy it; but I found none.

Therefore have I poured out mine indignation upon them; I have consumed them with the fire of my wrath: their own way have I recompensed upon their heads, saith the Lord God."

Judgment is coming down upon Americans because its Christians are unwilling to stand in the gap. They are not willing to engage in intercessory prayer for God to open doors in critical situations of national and international importance.

Promise Keeper's founder Coach Bill McCarthy states in the foreword of *What God Does When Men Pray* by William Carr Peel, that, "Through daily prayer and reading the Bible, Almighty God softens a man's heart, shapes his character, roots out sin in his life, and gives him direction and purpose. A like of prayer is foundational for a man who wants to run on all cylinders for God." [19]

MARCHING SHOULDER TO SHOULDER

We need to pray for our president. We need to get down on our knees and pray for him, that the Lord might appear to him in visions and speak to his heart to change the direction of this nation. Many times children speak to their parents in disrespectful ways. Why? Because we need to get down on our knees and pray and build a wall of righteousness by teaching them discipline. When we build up that wall of righteousness, we let them know that this mess cannot go on any longer. When we build up that wall of righteousness, we go marching shoulder to shoulder as a mighty people of God. Men of God, when we stand in the gap and build up that wall of righteousness, many of our men that do not have jobs will realize their place in life. They will realize God has called them to be the head of their family. They'll realize God has called them to be leaders in their community.

Thank God for single mothers, legal guardians, grandparents and all the other extended family members who have been standing in the gap for so many years. Thank God they have been standing in the gap and raising God's children and nurturing family members back to health and destiny. Yes, God is calling for us as a church to do His will, to not compromise, and to press on by walking through the doorway of destiny.

By pressing on we learn to walk through the doorway of destiny and be overcomers in life. We want to reach out and recognize our destiny and the new opportunity God has for us. First, we need to stand on our feet and claim it. We must make a commitment. Stand in the gap, even if the world is against you. Tell them, "I am willing to stand." Whether or not my family supports me. I will stand, whether or not my neighbors agree with me.

STANDING IN THE GAP FOR MAGIC JOHNSON

In 1991 the world-renown Los Angeles Lakers' basketball legend, Magic Johnson, announced at a TV press conference that a test for an insurance policy revealed he was infected with HIV, the AIDS virus. Cookie, Magic's wife, stood by his side and believed God in the face of impossibilities for his healing. Cookie said, "I honestly feel that the Lord is going to heal him and that we are going to live together forever and have more children and be happy."

She stood in the gap for her husband. After five years of taking his medication and standing on God's Word, doctors could not find any sign of the HIV virus in Johnson's blood. Magic still takes his medication and doctors credit his health status to the medicine only. Well, God works through miracles and medicine because without God none of these things would exist anyway.

Magic and Cookie are members of the West Angeles Church of God in Christ pastored by Bishop Charles Blake. The message of inner healing is best expressed in their lives through their own personal ministry to those who are wounded by AIDS. In 1991 they founded the Magic Johnson Foundation to financially support AIDS organizations that emphasize the message of AIDS education and prevention. Cookie stood in the gap for Magic and now they are both standing in the gap for the masses.

Whether they stab me in the back, I'm willing to stand in the gap as a man of God. For the only way to get our lost family members and friends through the doorway of destiny is by standing in the gap, and praying, fasting, and calling on the name of Jesus on their behalf. That is the spiritual warfare that brings about peace and inner healing.

11

INNER HEALING IN THE WILDERNESS

Isaiah 43:19: *"Behold, I will do a new thing; now it shall spring forth; shall ye not know it? I will even make a way in the wilderness, and rivers in the desert."*

The wilderness experience is a condition of existence, something that we all can relate to. If someone's testimony is that they've never seen trouble, they've never experienced the frustrations of life. Just wait until they've lived a little while longer, my brother, for one day they will go through the wilderness experience.

The wilderness experience is something every man of God, every human being can relate to—sooner or later. You cannot walk through the surrounding communities and not realize that there is a wilderness experience going on in our land.

Someone might ask, "What is the wilderness?" Let's define wilderness as an uncultivated, uninhabited region in our life. We experience the wilderness not just in the physical sense of walking through land dense with uncultivated vegetation, but also in areas spiritually that are uncultivated, and also through situations in life that need the hand of God to cultivate and change the situation.

Disease, divorce and death of a loved one are all examples of a wilderness experience. Financial debt and social economic deprivation is also a wilderness experience. Allen Sheffield writes in *Men to Men* that "the most important thing to do is live within your means. Do not spend more than you earn. The exercise of preparing a personal income statement will point out whether you are living beyond your means. You probably already know but putting it down on paper will help you see how much and where you can make cuts. [20]

Loneliness—when a single or a married brother feels he has no one to turn to, no one to talk to, no one to lean on—that is also part of the wilderness experience. The homeless have no place to sleep, nowhere to lay their heads, they are going through a wilderness experience.

But remember, Jesus came to make way in your wilderness to save, heal and deliver you to fulfill destiny! It doesn't matter where you are in life, whether you are rich or poor, this is something that we all must deal with. We don't have to go through some forty years of being out of the will of God to suffer a wilderness experience. We can deal with the reality of our everyday wilderness experiences in our own homes, jobs, and in our community and ministry and be right smack dab in the center of God's will. We can receive inner healing in our wilderness and rivers in our own deserts of life.

You Must Go Through Samaria

You can run, but you can't hide—for crime and violence occurs right around the corner and in front of some of the most faithful churches. There is a real wilderness in our cities, towns and villages that can't be ignored or else it will continue to grow wild and run rampant. There is a common denominator that faces everyone—you must deal with the wilderness before you reach your final destination in this journey called life.

Jesus put it like this, "You must go through Samaria." As we look at Scripture, one of the first things Jesus teaches us about wilderness experiences is that we must behold what God is doing even in the midst of the mess. We must pause and look at what God is doing. We look into our communities and we see various leaders saying, "I'm going to do this." We hear the politicians saying, "Since it is coming up near election, I will do this for the community, and I will make this change, and I will implement this plan." But we must stop, look, and listen to what the Lord has to say about the situation.

Every single day that God grants there are millions of men, women, boys and girls—sport lovers of every single race on God's good earth—who are encouraged and inspired by the life, legacy, and legend of the great Jackie Robinson, America's all-time baseball hero. He was also a messenger of inner healing and dignity. Jackie Robinson, a man of destiny, faith, and purpose, was despised, disenfranchised, and disrespected because of the color of his skin.

On April 15, 1947, Robinson played his very first major league baseball game at Ebbets Field in Brooklyn, New York, against the Boston Braves. Robinson went on to attain the honor of being named the highly coveted Rookie of the Year.

Proverbs 18:16 says, "*A man's gift maketh room for him, and bringeth him before great men.*" Well, Jackie Robinson's gift, his calling, his divine destiny—to play baseball in the major leagues and break the color line, and be an apostle of equality and justice—brought him the respect of world renown leaders such as the late civil rights leader, the Dr. Martin Luther King Jr.

Robinson signed that now historic contract with Brooklyn Dodger General Manager Branch Rickey, who told him, "We're tackling something big here, Jackie. If we fail, no one will try it again for twenty years...We're dealing with the right of any American to play baseball—the American game."

Prior to entering the Brooklyn Dodger clubhouse, Jackie played for the Montreal Royal. Prior to that, Robinson was the first athlete at UCLA to win a varsity letter in four different sports: baseball, basketball, football and track. He enrolled at UCLA in 1939. While at UCLA, Jackie met Rachel Isum who he married on Feb. 10, 1946. She played a major role in encouraging Jackie to fulfill the reason and purpose for which he was born: to be the first black man to break baseball's racial barriers.

Proverbs 18:22 affirms Jackie Robinson's choice in marriage: *"Who so findeth a wife, findeth a good thing, and obtaineth the favor of the Lord."*

When Robinson began to officially play for the Brooklyn Dodgers, he began receiving horrible death notes, such as one that read, "We have already got rid of several like you, one was found in the river just recently." Or, "Robinson, we are going to kill you if you attempt to enter the ball game at Crosley Field."

Robinson found his inner healing and essential wholeness by hitting a major home run in the opening game, which lead to a double victory, 10-3 and 14-4, for the Brooklyn Dodgers in the games against the Reds. April 15, 1997 marked the fiftieth anniversary of Jackie Robinson's historical entrance into the world of major league baseball. Jackie was able to be used by God in this manner because he was a man of destiny who knew how to find inner healing even in the wilderness of life.

BEHOLD, I WILL DO A NEW THING

My brothers, as we look at Scripture, the Word of God comes through to the prophet Isaiah that, "Behold I will do a new thing." God is trying to do a new thing in our midst even today. A lot of times we may feel threatened when we hear the word "new." Because one thing that stops the flow of God's anointing, one thing that stops His healing power, one thing that stops deliverance from the throne of God is tradition.

Yes, there are good traditions—our ancestry, the apostles and the writers of the Bible. But God wants us to move away from the traditions of the way things were done ten or twenty years ago. "He is saying, "Behold, I'm going to do a new thing."

This new thing is a matter of destiny and not foolishness. A new thing is only indicative of the fact that God wants to speak to the hearts of His people today. He wants to bring us to a higher level, to a higher dimension of His glory. God wants to bring us to a new threshold and move us in a new direction. He says, "Behold, I will do a new thing." Someone might wonder what "new thing" means. It means the sprouting forth and ushering in of God's power—in our homes, our jobs, our daily lives. This new experience can bring us out of the wilderness of life. It empowers us to run on to see what the end is going to be.

It's Me Standing in the Need of Prayer

We may experience God's grace coming down from the throne of glory as we intercede for someone's mother or father, but what we're really saying is, "It's me standing in the need of prayer." It becomes a new, fresh experience because there is nobody on the face of the earth just like you. God knows the number of hairs on your head. God knows every aspect about you. He knows everything about the chromosomes, genetic makeup, and DNA in your body.

There is nobody exactly like you. So when God does a new thing, He says, "I want to do something in your life." Nobody has yet heard the message coming through you. Someone else can give it, but it's not the same until you stand up and do what God has for you to do. God wants to get the majority that has been sitting back to rise up in faith and do a new thing. He wants to bring forth revival in the land—it begins in you and me.

Paul says in 2 Corinthians 5:17, *"If any man be in Christ, he is a new creature, old things are passed away. Behold, look and see, all things are become new."* It begins with the individual. God makes a new person. It's not good enough to just join the church. It's not good enough just to be baptized. Those are just symbols. We must be born again. We must be saved and forgiven of our sins.

We must become new. There are things that are holding and binding us. There are chains of bondage tied up all around us. Some people are in bondage to drugs, some are in bondage to alcohol and liquor, some are in bondage to cigarettes, some are in bondage to cursing, some are in bondage to lying. But the Lord says, "Behold, I want to make you a new creature."

OUR HELP COMES FROM THE LORD

So many people don't realize that God is the One who made us, He's even the One who woke us up this morning. Instead, they're running out to the soothsayer and they're listening to the psychics, but they need to run to Jesus.

Look to the hills from where our help comes. Our help doesn't come from the psychics, our help doesn't come from the astrologers, our help doesn't come from the soothsayers, our help doesn't come from the congregation—our help comes from the Lord, the Maker and Creator of heaven and earth. He can make all things new. Thank you, Jesus.

As we go through the wilderness and deserts of life, we must realize that God is watching over us. He has His angels of protection hovering above us, but there's something God wants us to do. He wants us to be able to pick up the Sword of the Spirit and chop down some of the debris, the branches and trees, and make a path for the Lord.

We're not the only people in the wilderness, but there are so many people who are hurting. Death, disease, divorce are all running rampant. Financial difficulty is going on in all major cities of the nation. We are in a wilderness experience. But God said that He will make a way out of no way, even in the wilderness, if we just learn to praise Him.

The Bible says God inhabits the praises of His people. When we praise God, even in the wilderness, He begins to chop down some trees. He begins to chop down some branches that are blocking our way to destiny. When we lift Him up and say "Hallelujah!" in the midst of the problem, He allows a path to be paved out in the wilderness that we might march on in the name of the Lord.

You cannot go forth with the flow of His anointing if you don't personally know the omnipotent One who is pouring down the oil of destiny. God wants to pour oil upon our heads, oil of His anointing, to prepare us to go forth and minister in the schools, the streets, the community. But He can't pour down the oil of destiny because we don't get down on our knees and pray.

It's not good enough for just the pastor to pray. It's not good enough for just the deacons or the trustees to pray. We all have to get down on our knees ourselves and call on the name of Lord in the midnight hour. God doesn't want us to strut our stuff and show ourselves off. God wants us to get in a prayer closet and call on His name.

Cry out to Him: "Jesus, I don't know how I'm going to make it through the wilderness. Trees and branches are falling down and blocking my way. Jesus, I need true inner healing. I need Your help. I need Your guidance. I need Your direction. I need Your protection. I need Your provision. Jesus, I need reviving from the stresses of life."

Larry Freeman writes in *Dealing with Stress: A Biblical Approach*, *"Jesus, our example was 'a man acquainted with grief'"* (Is. 53:3). Yet He endured all things, even facing death on the cross with joy. We can respond to stress in the same way. Stress can become a positive force in our lives, making us strong and giving us energy, developing our inner man and strong moral values, rather than discouraging and defeating us and causing us to be sick.

Dealing with stress means learning to be renewed in Christ. It means coming under certain disciplines, such as eating properly and getting enough exercise. It means conquering fears or phobias and learning to relax." [21]

You can pray this prayer: "Jesus, I need restoring. Jesus, I need Your help. Help me to spring forth, to leap forth in the power of the anointing." The Word says, "It's the anointing that destroys the yoke." The yoke of bondage that's over the drug addict's life. The yoke of bondage over the drunkard's life. The yoke of bondage over the liar's life, the yoke of bondage over the prostitute's life, the yoke of bondage over the pimp's life.

Such bondage can be destroyed only with the anointing that comes from the power of God working through His vessels—people. Then, we can stand up and say, "I've got a word from the Lord." It's not Rev. Mackey's word, it's not the choir's word, and it's not the church's word, but it's the word of the Lord.

We overcame the devil by the blood of the Lamb and by the word of our testimony." Do you have a testimony today? Do you have a story to tell? I don't know about you, but I have a story to tell. I've gone through the wilderness in the midnight hour. I've gone through the wilderness in the heat of the day, but I know the Lord is by my side. He will make a way.

He will make a way that leads to your personal doorway of destiny. God is doing a new thing. He wants us to have a new attitude. The Lord wants us to rise up and spring forth, leap forth, march on. The Bible says, "that I will even make a way in the wilderness, and rivers in the desert." Sometimes it seems like the stream of God's goodness begins to dry up in your life, that your prayers go up the ceiling and they bounce back down, but let me tell you that God can make a way out of no way.

My spiritual mind's eye goes back to a story in Exodus 17, after the children of Israel had left Egypt. They were wandering in the wilderness of sin, and the people said, "Moses, why did you bring us into the wilderness? There's no food here, no water, and it looks like God forgot about us."

They even wanted to murder Moses, to crucify him, but Moses got down on his knees and called out to God. The Lord said to Moses, "Moses! Pick up your rod and staff and go to the yonder rock and gather the children of Israel together. When you put your rod upon the rock, water will come out of the rock, even in the wilderness, even in the desert."

The water is symbolic of the move of the Holy Spirit. The Lord is telling us something similar: "Pick up your rod and hit the rock of trouble, pick up your rock through the Word of God, pick up your Sword of the Spirit, and speak the Word and water will come down from the portals of glory. Water that no man can stop, a river of living water."

Don't wait for someone to stir you up. Don't wait for someone to tell you to stand on your feet and praise God. Praise Him while you have a chance. Praise Him while the blood's still running warm through your veins. Give Him the glory, the honor, and the praise. When your back is up against the wall, give Him the glory.

When you can't pay your bills, give Him the glory. Give Him the honor. In the midst of death, give Him the glory. Give Him the honor in the midst of divorce. Give Him the glory, give Him the honor in the pressures of life. Soon and very soon God is going to look and see that you planted a seed and He will give you the increase. He will pour out His holy oil of inner healing for the torture and deeply troubled masculine soul.

If you learn to praise God in the wilderness, in the rough times of life, God will make a way that will lead you to civilization where doorways of destiny await you. You can walk through them and receive inner healing, deliverance, and restoration. The Lord Jesus Christ will grant you the inner healing you so desperately need.

God will make a way in your wilderness. You may be called to minister in the prisons, in the ghettos, and in the inner city crime-ridden areas. God will make a way in your wildness so you can fulfill your personal destiny.

Don't be afraid if God placed you in the wilderness to minister a message of hope and inner healing. If He put you there, that is part of your personal destiny to reach those people.

You can declare a word of faith, a word of hope, a word of love, a message of destiny— even in the wilderness. The mean streets of New York City are a real wilderness, but God needs His people to declare destiny in the Big Apple. The mean streets of Los Angeles are a real wilderness, but God needs some dedicated Christian soldiers who will stand for truth in that city of angels.

The mean streets of Detroit, Chicago and Washington, D.C. are real wilderness environments, but God is calling His people to declare divine destiny in those cities. God will make a clear cut-out path—a way in the wilderness—that leads to a doorway of destiny so we can change and influence a godless culture through the gospel of Jesus Christ. He desperately wants us to get involve in our communities and make a direct and lasting impact for His kingdom.

12

THE MINISTRY OF RECONCILIATION

God's Word tells us to seek first the kingdom of God, and all these things shall be added unto you. The reason why so many men are not reaping the benefits of a godly lifestyle is because seeking the kingdom of God is not first on their agenda. Many men are seeking the lust of the land instead of trying to live a kingdom lifestyle.

MEN OF PRAYER, PRAISE AND PURPOSE

We have been called out to be men of prayer, praise and purpose for the kingdom of God, for such a time as this. Amid our profane, perverse society, we have a distinct mandate from the Prime-Mover of divine destiny to restore the church to a prominent station of godly influence and spiritual power.

My brothers, both married and single, I am speaking of a purpose-filled position of authority that commands respect and demands a higher dimension of ethical and moral development and daily spiritual growth.

Galatians 6:1-3 bears witness to the extremely dire need to minister a message of faith, hope and restoration concerning our own personal predicaments, and moments of Christian crisis. This passage gives an accurate blueprint for spiritual growth and restoration that does not endorse, or emphasize a selfish philosophy of "me, myself and I" or a theology of super-spiritual arrogance. Galatians 6:1-3 firmly yet humbly states: *"Brethren, if man be overtaken in a fault, ye which are spiritual, restore such as one in the spirit of meekness; considering thyself, lest thou also be tempted. Bear ye one another's burdens, and so fulfill the law of Christ. For if a man think himself to be something, when he is nothing, he deceiveth himself."*

This fresh flamed revival of restoration and inner healing must first begin from the pulpit, the church officers, choirs, and entire church, and then it must be ushered out the door to touch the heart of the local community. This must be done to effectively reach and restructure the turbulent state of a truly disunited body of Christ, as well as win the lost for Christ.

How can today's church effectively reach the lost "third world" of America, the forgotten inner city, the sepulchered slum, the decaying ghetto of our nation, if we don't first take the time to separate ourselves in prayerful preparation and develop inner strength to face our own shortcomings.

Second Chronicles 7:14 says *"If my people, which are called by my name, shall humble themselves, and pray and seek my face, and turn from their wicked ways; then will I hear from heaven, and will forgive their sin, and will heal their land."*

The battered, broken, and bruised community is crying out for help, hope and hearing, like a hungry newborn baby in the midnight hour. Every television segment that emphasizes and exposes the lust of the land and the problems of this present age is a bloody outcry for help. Every slammin' and jammin' cut from a hard-core gangsta rapper, who wants to demean and disgrace women, is a vicious and violent cry for some serious help from the church.

Every single funeral for abused, confused, and misused young men and women, who are dead before their twentieth birthday because of the plight of peer pressure, dangerous drugs, and gruesome gang violence, is a tragic outcry for help from the church. In order to lead the lost through the doorway of destiny, the universal church must be restored and revived. This means that Baptist, Catholics, Methodist, Pentecostals, Independents, etc. will have to stop majoring in minors and get in the Spirit in order to hear more clearly the voice of God.

It's time to get right with God and for men to be real men of God. This must occur because the church is the only living organism and organization with the God-given ministry to reconcile the world to God.

Second Corinthians 5:18 says, *"And all things are of God, who hath reconciled us to himself by Jesus Christ, and hath given us the ministry of reconciliation."*

HEALING BROKEN RELATIONSHIPS

To reconcile means to adjust, to bring a broken relationship back to a state of harmony, unity and oneness. The ministry of reconciliation is the predestined mission and message of the church body. It's a message of inner healing sent straight from the Master concerning the crucial condition of the world. It is an essential aspect of the church's destiny and purpose to teach the lost by the example of a godly lifestyle.

The body of Christ must not be timid, afraid, or ashamed to say that if you live right, heaven belongs to you. If you don't, hell will be your eternal address. The apostle Paul said, *"I am not ashamed of the gospel of Jesus Christ for it is the power of God unto salvation"* (Rom. 1:16).

My brothers both married and single, in order for today's church to be effectively empowered for kingdom living in the last days we must not hide our light, our message. We must boldly minister these principles of kingdom living on a daily basis as stated in God's Word.

91

Second Corinthians 4:1-4 affirms this statement, *"Therefore seeing we have this ministry, as we have received mercy, we faint not; But have renounced the hidden things of dishonestly, not walking in craftiness, nor handling the word of god deceitfully; but by manifestation of truth commending ourselves to every man's conscience in the sight of God. But if our gospel he hid, it is hid to them that are lost. In whom the god of this world hath blinded the minds of them which believe not, lest the light of the glorious gospel of Christ, which is the image of God, should shine unto them."*

Politicians and other public officials won't live right if the priest of the Lord has a different moral code of ethical conduct. We are called as men of God to walk though our doorway of destiny, not the doorway of disgrace. God is able to deliver us if we only trust and obey His voice.

The masses of people who populate the planet have lost hope in the church, yet when trouble comes they innately cry out "Oh God!" and turn to the blessed assurance of their youth. It is a lame excuse to say to the world, "Well don't put your trust in the church, trust in God," when we are His vessels here on earth. It is true that we must trust in God for direction concerning our personal destiny, but integrity and a personal responsibility to live right must not be thrown under the rug. Paul was able to say "follow me as I follow Christ," because Paul had his priorities straight.

We all have sinned and fallen short of the glory of God (Rom. 3:23), but we don't have to stay in a pig pen and give worthless excuses. Like the prodigal son we need to come to our senses and make the journey back home. Now is the time to rise up and be the church triumphant. We must not be holier than thou in our demeanor, but we must be genuinely concerned about the plights of others. The church is God's mouthpiece, His trombone to declare what divine destiny is regarding every aspect of life.

GOD IS CALLING MEN TO BE SOLID ROLE MODELS

This is extremely important because the world needs solid role models who cannot be bought and who will not sell out on the Savior. Our youth need some destiny dealers who can save their future through the power of God. The church must develop these strong Spirit-filled role models from their own ranks. Doctors, lawyers, policemen, physicians, pastors, Christian rappers, teachers, college professors, etc., must be developed from our own ranks.

The church has inherited the needed components to change society through the life, death, and resurrection of Jesus Christ. In a real sense God has given the church the authority to stop the madness. Our ability to stop the madness is found in the power of influence in terms of our daily lifestyle.

Let us check our own church rolls because many of the men I minister to in prison are forgotten male members of local churches. In many cases they get in trouble because of the absence of strong Christian role models.

As men of God if we constantly dance to the beat of the world, drink wine and liquor, smoke, curse, fuss, and fight, then go to church on Sunday to praise the Lord in the beauty of holiness, then how in the world can we ask our embattled youth not to do drugs, crime, and violence. They're following in our footsteps. It is the actual practice of biblical principles in the home that creates an environment and atmosphere that promotes true Christian progress.

13

INNER HEALING FOR SINGLE MEN

When a man is single it is an excellent time for him to get close to God. Paul wrote one-third of the New Testament and traveled far and wide preaching the gospel of Jesus Christ as a single man deeply committed to God.

The state of singlehood is a time for true inner healing and essential wholeness prior to getting into a serious relationship that could lead to marriage. In other words, as a single man now is the time to get right with God, before obtaining the responsibility of not only your own body, but that of a wife and children.

SINGLE, SAVED AND SATISFIED

If you already have a child, are divorced, or are in a tight situation, God still cares. He wants the single man to discover wholeness through the power of the Holy Spirit. All men—married, single, or divorced—must pray this following prayer for wholeness:

"Holy Spirit, breathe on me. Holy Spirit, breathe in me. Holy Spirit, breathe through me. You are my Source of inner healing. Help me be the single man You called me to be. Help me be responsible and effective in all that I do. Let all that I do be done only for Your glory. Help me be a man. Lord, please help me be a ` true man of God who walks in Your footsteps and is an imitator of Jesus Christ. Help me process the pain, problems, and predicaments I face daily. Help me love my wife. Help me love my daughter. Help me love my son. Help me love my parents. Help me make the right decisions and not go down any wrong paths. Help watch who I spend my time with. Help me build healthy and non-toxic relationship. For through Christ I can do all things."

As single, married, re-married, and divorced men we need to truly catch the vision of victory that the Holy Spirit is our inner healing. No matter what hurt. No matter what pain. No matter what trail or tribulation. God can breathe on your circumstance of total failure and make your life a lasting success and testimony of His mighty power.

God can teach you how to love without lust. God can teach you how to remain sexually pure, even if you've lost your virginity once or a thousand times over. God can give you what Edwin Cole calls "the glory of sex."

The "glory of sex" is when a single man or woman repents of having sex outside of marriage and abstains from sexual intercourse until they are officially married. Only God can do that. For the shedding of blood from the women's hymen represents a blood covenant, a blood contract, or agreement, which is only ordained by God for marriage.

THE HOLY SPIRIT, OUR SOURCE OF INNER HEALING

John 14:26-27 says, *"But the Comforter, which is the Holy Ghost, whom the Father will send in My Name, He shall teach you all things, and bring all things to your remembrance, whatsoever I have said unto you. Peace I leave with you, My peace I give unto you; not as the world giveth, give I unto you. Let not your heart be troubled, neither let it be afraid."*

Bow Our Spirit in Submission to His Will

Quite often we can actually feel the Holy Spirit as our Source of inner healing. His presence, moving in our midst, touches our heart, spirit and soul, in a miraculous way as we lifted up our hands in adoration. We bow our spirits in submission to His perfect and holy will.

Sometimes men will withhold their worship and praise as though they're begrudging the Holy Spirit. But the Bible says, "Grieve not the Holy Spirit." Many times we talk with fellow brothers in Christ about God the Father, and we talk about Jesus His Son, but we ignore the work of the Holy Spirit, the Comforter. As men in drastic need of meaning, we need the Holy Spirit working in our lives each and every day. We need the Holy Spirit in our homes, our jobs, and in every decision we make. We need the influence, and the direction, and the guidance of the Holy Spirit.

He Is the Comforter

What is the power and work of the Holy Ghost? In verse 26, Jesus says, *"But the Comforter."* The Comforter, the One who is called alongside to help us. The One who is called to give us guidance. The One who is called to give us assistance. The One who comes in the midst of our turmoil, our pain. The One who comes in the midst of our heartache and disease.

Part of the power and work of the Holy Spirit is that He is the Comforter. No matter what you're going through, the Holy Ghost is your Comforter. Your mother or father may have recently passed away, your wife may have left you or maybe you're having trouble with your son. Someone close to you might be strung out on drugs or in prison. But the Holy Spirit is still your Comforter, your total Source of inner healing.

He Has Not Forgotten About You

The Holy Spirit, our Source of inner healing, comes to bring comfort in the midst of your pain, comfort in the midst of your wounds, and comfort in the midst of your heartache. No matter what you're going through, the Holy Spirit wants to bring comfort to the comfortless. If you're going through hard times and just don't feet at ease, you don't know what to do, you're trying to find direction, the Holy Spirit wants to bring calm.

HE IS A TEACHER

Not only is the Holy Spirit a Comforter, but He is also an excellent Teacher. If you need to get close to God, you need to get close to His Holy Spirit. We need the Holy Spirit to begin to work, and to move more effectively in life because the Holy Spirit is a teacher.

If you don't feel really familiar with the Bible even though you read it regularly, maybe you don't get a clear understanding of what it is saying, then you need to ask the Holy Spirit to give you guidance and direction.

When you read a particular verse on your own, you might read, "The Lord is my Shepherd I shall not want," and it will just be surface knowledge. But when you ask the Holy Spirit to give you some understanding, you'll read "The Lord is my shepherd," and you'll begin to personalize that and realize that everywhere you go, the great Shepherd is watching over . It'll become a totally new and exciting revelation to you. When you ask the Holy Spirit to reveal things to you, He will bring you into all truth.

If there is something you don't know how to deal with, the Holy Spirit can show you. Maybe you'll pray, "Lord, I don't know how to deal with finances. Holy Spirit, show me how." The Holy Spirit will send someone into your life who knows how to deal with finances; a pastor or friend who will give you guidance and show you how to make up a budget and live within your financial means.

If you don't know how to deal with peer pressure or a bully, the Holy Spirit can show you the best way to deal with that particular person or persons. He will teach you how to stand up for what is right. The Holy Spirit will teach you all things.

If someone is abusing you and you've been in that situation too long, the Holy Spirit will teach you all things and show you how to exit that situation.

THE HOLY SPIRIT HELPS YOU REMEMBER WHAT JESUS SAID TO YOU

The Holy Spirit will teach you all things, not just the things you think are spiritual, but the things of life, the issues of life that you don't consider spiritual. When you feel like cursing at somebody, the Holy Spirit will teach you all things. When you're ready to hit somebody because they called you everything but a child of God, the Holy Spirit will teach you teach you how to conduct yourself.

We're talking about the power and the work of the Holy Spirit that brings inner healing for the wounded masculine soul. The Holy Spirit is here to comfort you and heal your deepest wounds and worst scars. You might be bleeding right now, but He's here with some bandages and ointment to bring healing to your wounded soul.

The Holy Spirit will bring to our remembrance whatever Jesus has said to us. That means we need to have a little talk with Jesus and tell Him about our troubles.

It also means that if we don't talk to Jesus, there is nothing that the Holy Spirit will bring to our remembrance. You put something into the computer, then you can retrieve information. If you don't put information into the computer, you can't pull anything out.

If we want the power and the work of the Holy Spirit, our Source of inner healing, to flow in our lives, we have to pray. We must not have just a monologue with God where we're doing all the talking and telling Him everything we want. Rather, we need to get quiet before God and let Him speak to our hearts.

So if we talk to Jesus, the Holy Spirit will bring back to our remembrance things that Jesus said to us. When was the last time Jesus talked to you? You better let Him talk to you in the shower or while you're brushing your teeth. Let Him speak to you when you're washing up. Let Him talk to you when you're down on your knees. Let Him talk to you as you're driving your car. Let Him talk to you while you're walking up and down at your job. Let Him talk to you, my brother, everywhere you go. Let the presence of the Lord permeate your being, your spirit, your soul and body so everyday you can begin to hear the voice of Jesus more clearly.

PEACE IN THE MIDST OF THE STORM

Peace. I like that word. If anybody asks you what is in a healing, it is peace. When Jesus brings peace to your mess, that's inner healing. When Jesus brings you peace despite the storm that's enveloped you, that's inner healing. That peace might be a word of hope that He's going to bring you out of the storm. But if you have that peace that passes all understanding, then you've got inner healing.

Jesus says this peace "I leave with you." Want to know what this peace is? Want to know what this inner healing is? The Holy Ghost, He is a Person. Jesus left Him with us you. He is a Spirit. God is a Spirit and they that worship Him, must worship Him in spirit and in truth. This Spirit is peace, love, and joy in the Holy Ghost. This peace, the Holy Ghost, I leave with you.

The peace that the world gives is limited and conditional. They might stop fighting a war or stop trying to kill each other for a little while, but then it will begin again.

Jesus says, "My peace, the Holy Spirit, I give unto you." He says, "Let not your heart be troubled, neither be afraid." So no matter what you're going through, let not your heart be troubled or neither be afraid because you have the peace of God. You have the power and the presence of the Holy Spirit working in your life. You have the God of inner healing for men, women, boys and girls, working within you and there is nothing that you cannot overcome.

CALLED FOR EXCELLENCE

Look at the life of the apostle Peter. Peter denied Christ three times. Peter saw Jesus in the distance walking on the water and got off of the ship to walk on the water himself—before he started sinking.

Many of us focus only on the point that he began to sink, but Peter did walk on water. When he took his eyes off Jesus, he began to sink. If you want to stay in the flow and the move of the Holy Spirit, don't take your eyes off Jesus. Don't focus on what a person is doing, but keep your eyes on Jesus.

"Press toward the mark of the high calling which is in Christ Jesus." Realize that you're called for excellence. Keep your eyes on Jesus. Satan tried to sift Peter like wheat, but one thing I like about Peter is that he kept on trying. Neither you nor I may reach the one-hundred mark each and every day, but if we just keep trying, God will bless that. Even in the midst of all of Peter's failures, he kept pressing on to do his best.

When they tried to carry Jesus off to be crucified, Peter stood up and cut off one of the guard's ears. Jesus, in essence said, "Hey, this is ordained to be, I'm going to die and rise again in three days, leave them alone." And He instantaneously healed the guard's ear. Peter was trying to stand up for his Lord in his own way. He was wrong many times, but he tried.

Even though we might be wrong sometimes, God knows our heart. When Jesus rose from the dead, He said, "Go tell My disciples, and Peter, that I have risen." Talk about the power and the work of the Holy Spirit as our Source of inner healing, just take a look at a wounded life in the man of Peter. What a messed-up life, but the Holy Spirit began to mold him and look what Peter ended up accomplishing for the kingdom.

During Pentecost, people from all different parts of the world were outside the building witnessed those who were in the upper room speaking in their own language. Who is it that preaches the first sermon in the new Christian church? Peter.

I share that with you to give you an example of the power and the work of the Holy Spirit. No matter what you have done, God has a plan for your life. Remember what Jesus said to you in your times of personal prayer and private Bible study. If you are single, now is your time to draw close to God and He will draw close to you.

COME, YE DISCONSOLATE

1.) Come, ye disconsolate, where'er ye languish—Come to the mercy-seat, fervently kneel; Here bring your wounded hearts, here tell your anguish: Earth has no sorrow that heav'n cannot heal. (Come, Ye Disconsolate, Verse 1, Thomas Moore, *The New National Baptist Hymnal*, National Baptist Publishing Board, Nashville, Tenn., July 1980, p. 228.)

14

OVERCOMING TEMPTATION

Hebrews 4:15 says, *"For we have not an high priest which cannot be touched with the feeling of our infirmities; but was in all points tempted like as we are, yet without sin."*

Our High Priest, Jesus Christ, is the risen Redeemer of the lost souls who was literally touched by the feeling of our infirmities. When my father died an early death due to colon cancer, Jesus was touched by the feeling of his infirmity. When a man is living off of food stamps and trying to find a job every single day without any success, Jesus is touched by the feeling of his infirmity. When a brother is dying of AIDS and is an outcast to his so-called friends, Jesus is touched by the feeling of his infirmity.

Jesus is deeply moved by our pain; He has the provision for our healing. The finished work of the crucified and risen Savior, Jesus Christ, provides the inner healing as well as the physical healing that we need.

Not only does Jesus understand the feeling of our infirmity, Jesus also understands a whole lot about enduring temptation as man, who was also God.

The Son of God took on human flesh. He was tempted just like everyone else. Jesus was tempted to have sex with women who were not his wife, his bride, the church. Jesus was tempted to steal. Jesus was tempted to kill. He had to be tempted, and yet without sin in order for the Scriptural record to be true. Long before Jesus taught the golden rule to the disciples, He was tempted to drink booze with the boys. Whatever horrible sin that could be mentioned, Jesus was tempted with its equivalent during His day.

The Bible clearly says that Jesus "was in all points tempted like as we are, yet without sin." That is the very reason why we can sing: "Jesus knows all about our troubles. He will guide us until the day is through. There's not a friend like the lowly Jesus no not one. No not one."

It is extremely important for men to know that Jesus is a Savior who can relate to our everyday temptations, yet He gives men the key to endure and not yield to temptation. Everyone will be tempted, enticed by evil, just like Jesus was, but Jesus shows men how to receive the inner healing and essential wholeness that is necessary to endure temptation.

James 1:12 states, *"Blessed is the man that endureth temptation: for when he is tried, he shall receive the crown of life, which the Lord hath promised to them that love him."*

As men in need of divine inner healing and essential wholeness from the Holy Spirit, we must realize that we are called to endure temptation. In fact, the Christian cannot receive the crown of life without correctly choosing the God-given option to endure temptation.

Quite naturally the man who deeply desires the divine touch of the Father's healing hand would ask how did Jesus endure temptation, everyday enticement of evil in the world that surrounds you. James 1:2, 4 says, *"My brethren, count it all joy when ye fall in diverse temptations. Knowing this, that the trying of your faith worketh patience...But let patience have he perfect work, that ye may be perfect and entire wanting nothing."*

God desires for men to rejoice in the times of temptation and enticement to do wrong, because these are the very moments where He molds and lays a firm foundation for men to learn to do the right thing. They'll discover they love God more than liquor, women, or drugs. Jesus calls men to find joy by enduring temptation, not given in to negative peer pressure from our friends and colleagues.

Enduring temptation always leads to inner healing. The tempting, the worldly enticement, the trying of our faith brings an inner strength better known today as patience. There is a clear process of inner healing and essential wholeness that brings a man from the point of always yielding to temptation to the point in which he endures and stands up for what he believes. God is calling on men to come closer to the foot of the cross in the time of temptation. God is not the tempter, the devil is, and he especially uses your own lust as the bait to draw you into the death ring of temptation.

James 1:13-15 clearly backs this point up when it declares, "*Let no man say when he is tempted, I am tempted of God: for God cannot be tempted with evil, neither tempteth he any man: But every man is tempted, when he is drawn away of his own lust, and enticed. Then when lust hath conceived, it bringeth forth sin: and sin, when it is finished, bringeth forth death.*"

Yet God tells men to rejoice in the time of great temptation for it is His boot camp to teach men the real meaning of wholeness and holiness through the process of enduring temptation. God uses the time of temptation in which the enemy has a field day in the backyard of men's own lust as a God-ordained opportunity for men to turn to Christ. Then, they can crucify the control of the flesh and yield to the work of the Holy Spirit.

We all know that Jesus was tempted just like we are today, but how did He endure and not yield to temptation? As men it is drastically important and imperative that we learn lessons and glean the truth from Jesus' classic examples in the time of temptation.

Every single temptation and enticement of one's own lust is a temptation that is common to man.

There is nothing new under the sun. There is no sin that God has never heard of. God desires men to endure temptation in order to overcome the death grip of the enticement of evil.

The children of Israel wandering in the wilderness for forty years is a classic example; God delivered them out of slavery and bondage in Pharaoh's Egypt under the God-ordained leadership of Moses. God parted the Red Sea for the Israelites and literally drowned Pharaoh's army. But their inner lusts to murmur and to complain kept them out of the Promised Land. There is no temptation that is uncommon to man, there is nothing new under the sun—sin is sin.

While the Book of James clearly teaches that God never tempts us, the Holy Spirit may at times lead us into a wilderness experience where we are tempted. But hold fast to the confession of your faith during that time of temptation and that will make all the difference. Just like it did when Jesus was tempted by the devil in His own wilderness experience.

Matthew 4:1-11 states: *"Then was Jesus led up of the Spirit into the wilderness to be tempted of the devil. And when he had fasted forty days and forty nights, he afterward an hungered. And when the tempter came to him, he said, If thou be the Son of God, command that these stones be made bread. But he answered and said, It is written, Man shall not live not by bread alone, but by every word that proceedeth out of the mouth of God. Then the devil taketh him up into the holy city, and setteth him on a pinnacle of the temple. And saith unto him, If thou be the Son of God, cast thyself down: for it is written, He shall give his angels charge concerning thee: and in their hands they shall bear thee up, lest at any time thou dash thy foot against a stone Jesus said unto him, It is written again, Thou shalt not tempt the Lord thy God. Again, the devil taketh him up into an exceeding high mountain, and showeth him all the kingdoms of the world, and the glory of them; And saith unto him, All these things will I give thee, if thou wilt fall down and worship me. Then saith Jesus unto him, Get thee hence, Satan: for it is written, Thou shalt worship the lord thy God, and him only shalt thou serve. Then the devil leaveth him, and behold, angels came and ministered unto him."*

Jesus Christ, the Son of God, who came to earth in the form of man, fully understands what it means to be tempted by the devil. You would think that the Holy Spirit would have led Jesus to some place other than the wilderness. But Jesus wants to minister to you in your personal wilderness just as the angels ministered to Him in His.

To the man addicted to promiscuity, Jesus wants to minister to him in his wilderness. That man may think it's all fun and games and that there's nothing wrong with putting a few more notches in your grand prized trophy belt, but God wants you to use that same energy to reach lost souls for His kingdom.

Jesus is calling you to the altar of real repentance. Instead of putting more notches in your belt, Jesus wants to revolutionize your life and give you a new sense of purpose, clear direction, and divine destiny for the new millennium.

To the man deceived by the lie of homosexuality, Jesus is calling him to receive divine deliverance from his personal wilderness. Same-sex relationships are a camouflage for the brokenness of a past that has plagued your present and threatens your future. God loves you, but He clearly hates the homosexual lifestyle, just as much as He clearly hates the heterosexual sin of sleeping with every woman possible. Or the sin of masturbating—wasting the seed as an outlet and release.

All three are dangerous perversions and lies against God's perfect plan for love-making between a husband and wife. God also has a perfect plan for the single man—to be made whole deep within and without, by seeking God first and being made complete in everyday life through a solid and steadfast relationship with Christ.

The bottom line is that sin is sin, and God hates it all. Use of crack, cocaine, reefers, weed, marijuana, etc., as well as alcohol will only distort reality, ruin life and deeply hurt families. Endure the temptation. Don't give in. You can have the victory over it all.

No matter what the sin, the key is that the blood of Jesus can wipe it away and put you on the road to a new life. No matter what the temptation, God will never give up on you. The worst con artist, thief, murderer, hate-monger, etc., in the world does not have to die in their sin.

There is healing for every wounded soul. You can receive forgiveness from the Lord and your life can be reformed realistically. Moses was a murderer, but God ministered to his soul on the backside of the dessert and prepared him to become a deliverer of His people. Jesus is married to the backslider, so your private sin is not too much for His amazing grace.

God wants men simply to be open and honest, vulnerable and unashamed so He can heal their broken, battered, and bruised souls. His grace is amazing, but it is not a cheap grace. Yes, His grace is so amazing because He actually does see man's need to be made whole.

The key lesson Jesus teaches us from His wilderness experience is to endure and overcome the temptation by utilizing the strategy of speaking God's Word with deep fervor and solid conviction in the face of the tempter. You will finally come to the place where His angels minister to you after you have endured and overcame your own particular temptation experience in the wilderness of life.

Even when you have endured a fiery trail of temptation, God will minister inner healing and essential wholeness to your tortured soul. God has promised you a crown of life for enduring temptation because you love Him more. Your life has a new focus, so speaking and living God's Word and truly trusting in Him completely is the key to endure in your time of temptation.

15

Stir Up the Gift Within

Paul writes in 2 Timothy 1:1-7, to his son in ministry. Timothy is one of the first young pastors in the early church of our Lord and Savior, Jesus Christ. God accomplished a marvelous work in this young man's life. Paul had stepped in to be a surrogate father to Timothy.

"Paul, an apostle of Jesus Christ by the will of God, according to the promise of life which is in Christ Jesus, to Timothy my dearly beloved son, grace, mercy and peace from God the Father, and from Christ Jesus our Lord. I thank God, whom I serve from my forefathers with a pure conscience, that without ceasing I have remembrance of thee in my prayers night and day, greatly desiring to see thee, being mindful of thy tears, that I may be filled with joy. When I call to remembrance the unfeigned faith that is in thee, which dwelt first in my grandmother Lois, and thy mother Eunice; and I am persuaded that in thee also. Wherefore I put thee in remembrance that thou stir up the gift of God, which is in thee by the putting on of my hands. For God hath not given us the spirit of. fear, but of power, and of love, and of a sound mind."

When Paul writes his opening greeting to Timothy, notice he greets him with three words: *grace, mercy* and *peace*. Paul uses this greeting only when he writes to pastors. When he writes to the churches, he says, "Grace and mercy." Paul realized these pastors needed the peace of God to prevail in their lives because there were problems going on in dealing with people.

A FATHER IN MINISTRY

In our walk with the Lord, we need fathers in ministry. A father in the ministry is a pastor who watches out for your soul. He makes sure you are spiritually equipped with the Word of God. He knows that Satan will try to come against you, so in his teaching and preaching, he makes sure you're equipped with the things you need to overcome the devil.

THE ROLE OF A LEADER

As Christians, we must learn that not only must the pastor stir up the gift of God within him, but members of the church must also individually and collectively stir up the gift of God within them. God has a gift He has given each of us. God has a calling that is upon your life and He wants you to fulfill that gift. He wants you to fulfill that calling upon your life.

The Book of 2 Timothy is mandatory reading for all pastors, but it's also mandatory reading for all Christians who are serious about the work of the Lord. It's not a book for those who want to be lightweights in the gospel. It's not a book for those who don't want to make an impact on society. It's a book for those who want to make a difference, who want to bring about a change in society. Paul tells us how to stir up the gift of God within each of us.

A GIFT TO REMEMBER

Proverbs 18:16 says that a man's gift will make room for him, and bring him before great men. The Greek word used in that verse is *mattan*, which means a present, a gift, something to give, a reward. There is a gift, a present God has given to you and He wants you to share that gift with someone else.

When I was at Christ Chapel headquarters in Nigeria, I was returning one morning from a church service and saw some young people making signs and banners to hang up for an upcoming meeting. Instantly in my spirit I thought about that Scripture, that a man's gift will make room for him and bring him before great men. We must present our God-given talents, skills and abilities as gifts unto the Lord. Those young men and women were drawing and utilizing their artistic talents as a gift unto the Lord.

A FEAST FOR THE PALETTE

I was talking with my brothers after dinner and I shared with them that the food was so good in Africa. It was so good that it made your tongue rise up and slap your brains out. The men and women who prepared the food used their cooking talents, skills, and abilities as gifts unto God. Not everybody has the gift to cook that type of good food. Therefore, they cannot present it as a gift. You taste some food that somebody else prepared and you want to push the plate away. But when they have the skills, talents and abilities to cook, they've got an anointing to cook. Not only will your soul be blessed, but your stomach and taste buds will be blessed, too!

My pastor, the late Rev. Arthur Mackey Sr., every year would always prepare "the pastor's stew." He would get out his big cooking pot and fill it with potatoes, onions, carrots, string beans, different types of meat, the best sauce, and a little bit of this and that. He would cook it over a low fire. He'd always say, "Don't turn up the fire too high because we don't want it to burn at the bottom. If it burns at the bottom and you begin to stir it, it will stir up a bad taste and nobody will want to come back and get any more."

So, there was a young man who would always stand at the pot and stir the stew. That young man is the one who wrote this book. I would stand there and stir that pot of stew and in my spirit God

111

was showing me that we have to stir up the gift of God that is within us.

THE MAIN INGREDIENT

Within each of us there is not just potatoes, string beans, carrots, different types of meat. Instead, there are callings and gifts that God has placed in His congregation. We have to stir up those things. We cannot put all of the responsibility on the pastor. The pastor must share the vision, but we must go out and make that vision a reality.

We must take the Word that God has given us and apply it to real-life situations. We must apply it to the hard times we endure, apply it to our situations and predicaments and our present existence.

God may have given you a gift to teach, preach, sing, witness, draw, write, counsel, run, dance, work with children, counsel married couples, counsel divorced people, counsel the bereaved. Whatever the gift, it was God Who revealed it to you in the midnight hour or in those weak times or during a quiet prayer time. He wants you to stir up that gift within you, stir up that anointing. Don't let it burn up because the fire is burning. Keep it stirred up, keep it flowing, keep it growing, keep it going for Jesus.

GOD WANTS TO USE YOU

Don't let that gift remain dormant. God wants to use you. He wants to use your voice to sing. He wants to use your voice to witness. He wants to use your hands to prepare meals. He wants to use your hands to draw great signs and murals. He wants to use your hands to make great statues, something that displays the gospel of Jesus.

In 2 Timothy, we realize Paul has a spiritual assignment from God. That spiritual assignment is to help Timothy remember—because sometimes you have to remember where God brought you from.

Acts 16 gives us some background about this young man Timothy: *"Then came he to Derby and to Listra,"* talking about the apostle Paul. "And behold a certain disciple..." So we know that before Timothy became a great pastor, he was a disciple. He was a follower of Christ. So many folks want to go straight to the big positions, but the way to go up in Christ is to go down on your knees, to be a servant.

It says, "he was a disciple named Timothus... the son of a certain woman who was a Jewess, and believed she was a Christian." She was a Christian Jew. "But his father was a Greek." So, we have a problem here. Knowing Timothy is a disciple, many of the Christians who were also Jews did not want to accept him because his father was Greek. This was an interracial child and some folks had problems with Timothy coming in and trying to do the work of the Lord. It was a racism of sorts. There was discrimination of sorts occurring, both in the physical and in the religious sense.

NATIONALITY DOESN'T MAKE A DIFFERENCE

The fact that Timothy's father was Greek should not have mattered at all, but it did matter in the hearts and minds of many of the men and women, who really didn't have themselves right with God. *"Which was well reported by the brethren that were in Listra in Iconium. Him would Paul have to go forth with him, and took and circumcised him, because of the Jews which were in those quarters, for they all knew that his father was a Greek,"* (Acts 16:2).

Paul said, in essence, "Instead of me fussing with everybody, I'm just going to take Timothy to be circumcised because the gospel needs to be preached, whether it is a Jew or a Greek. In order for the gift of God to be stirred up in us, there are some things we have to circumcise. There are some things we have to cut off. There are some things we have to allow God to cut away. It might hurt and be painful, but then the gift can come forth."

COMMITTED TO THE CAUSE

First, you must remember to pray. You must have a life committed to prayer. Don't take prayer lightly, but be serious about prayer and realize that God is not a being we talk about. He is an everlasting God, He is an awesome God, and He is the almighty God who can transform our lives.

Secondly, not only must we remember to pray, but Paul says in verse four, "Greatly desiring to see thee, and being mindful of thy tears." He knew that Timothy would pray and he would cry. All of the hardships that he was experiencing, Paul had to tell him, "Grace, mercy and peace."

Paul spoke the peace of God in life. In the midst of his tears, and in the midst of his struggles, Paul realized what was going on in Timothy's life. He said, "You've got to remember where God has brought you from, that you may be filled with joy."

FILLING THE VOID

"When I call to remembrance the unfeigned faith that is in thee which dwelt first in thy grandmother Lois." Paul doesn't mention Timothy's father the Greek. This is written many years after the earlier account in Acts. Maybe Timothy's father is now dead, I don't know. But I do know that the Scripture clearly lets us know that in verse 2, Paul calls him, "Timothy, my dearly beloved son."

Whatever is missing in your life, God will fill that void. There may be someone who has lost a child, someone who has experienced a divorce, someone whose mother or father is gone. There's a void in your life, but God, through His awesome presence and power, will fill that void. There is no one who will ever be your mother, no one who will ever be your father, and no one who ever be your son or daughter. Only God can fill that void in your life.

What God wants to do is fill that void with the gift that He has placed in you. As you utilize that gift, you're utilizing the training you got from your mother or father. If you were a Christian, you're utilizing the training, even far greater than that which God has already placed in your life. God is calling us to stir up the gift that is within us. He's calling us to stir up the gift that will fill the void that is in our lives.

Verse five says, "I call to remembrance that unfeigned faith." Paul is calling us to remember our heritage of faith. Not only does he call us first of all to pray, because prayer is one of the foundations of revival, but he's calling us to remember our rich heritage of faith. That is the other way we stir up the gift of God within us—by remembering to pray.

By remembering our rich heritage of faith, we realize the church is much larger than we could ever imagine. We also realize there are brothers and sisters all across Africa, America, Asia, Europe, and India who are worshipping God in spirit and in truth.

Not only that, the church also includes the dead in Christ. It also includes all those in the New Testament church who died in the faith such as: Paul, Timothy, Matthew, Mark, Luke and John. It includes the Old Testament believers as well such as: Elijah, Isaiah, Habakkuk, Nahum, Zephaniah, and saints like Moses and David. When we begin to look at our rich Christian heritage, we realize it includes great men and women of God throughout the ages in every walk of life.

We have a family; we're not in this thing alone. Not only are we called to stir up the gift of God within us, but also we are supposed to stir up the gifts within our brothers and sisters in the ministry. God is calling us to stir up the gift of God within us.

The first point is to remember to pray, if you want to stir up the gift of God. Second, remember your rich Christian heritage of faith, if you want to stir up the gift of God within you.

THE HOLY SPIRIT CAN'T BE CONTROLLED

Rev. Bernice King, daughter of the late civil rights leader Dr. Martin Luther King Jr., said that "The Holy Spirit cannot be controlled by us; instead, the Holy Spirit controls us. When something controls us, it means something has gotten deep inside us. That's why all throughout the Book of Acts, it says that the apostles were filled with the Holy Spirit, not that they had the Holy Spirit." When you're filled with the Holy Spirit no problem is too difficult to handle, no burden too difficult to bear, no illness too difficult to heal. That's why we can have the Holy Spirit and still not have real power. But when we are filled with the Holy Spirit, we have power that can take on the world."

BURN IT UP

Have you ever seen a tree when it is dried out and begins to catch fire? Then another tree is ignited and flames begin to spread through the forest like wild fire. They don't know how to stop it from consuming all the grass and tress. My Bible tells me that our God is a consuming fire. That's what God wants us to do.

In fact, the word *gift* in 2 Timothy 1:6 means *"to snatch, terminate, consume."* God wants to give you a gift that will consume you. God wants to give you a gift that will bum up everything not holy in your life. God wants to give you a gift that will bum up everything not right in your life. God wants to give you a gift for everything that's not righteous in your life.

THERE'S A PURPOSE FOR THE GIFT

God gives you this gift and its purpose is to consume everything that is not right in you—to purge it out, to purify you, to bring sanctification into your life. If God has called you to sing, sing and give God all the praise. As you play those drums, as you work on those tapes, stir up the gift. Day by day, as you stir up the gift within you, it consumes you. It puts a deep desire in you to serve Him even more.

But now, since you're using your gift, it consumes you. You have your mind on the things of God and the work of the ministry. You might be fixing food for a church function and as you cook, you realize you're ministering. As you prepare a sauce, you're ministering. As you drive the van, you're ministering. As you carry the pastor's briefcase, you're ministering. As you go out on the streets and witness, you realize you're ministering. You're stirring up the gift of God within you.

ABIDE IN THE GIFT

You have the gift because God laid His hands on you. You could have been avoided, you could have died, but you're here right now. You have to stir up that gift. You have to use that gift. Your gift will make room for you. Your gift will kick doors down for you, and your gift will consume you. Anything that's not right, it will bum it up, if you just use the gift. If you flow in the anointing, if you walk in your calling, if you realize God chose you—you have stirred up the gift.

TELL SOMEONE ABOUT JESUS

God is saying, instead of going that route, "Let My consuming fire move in your life." "For God so loved the world that He gave His only begotten Son that whosoever believeth in Him should not perish but have everlasting life."

16

Inner Healing In Troubled Times

P salm 138:7 states that, *"Though I walk in the midst of trouble, thou wilt revive me: thou shalt stretch forth thine hand against the wrath of mine enemies, and thy right hand shall save me."*

In 1999 my father, the Rev. Dr. Arthur Mackey Sr., was diagnosed with colon cancer that eventually spread to his liver. My father was the highly esteemed pastor of Mount Sinai Baptist Church in Roosevelt, New York, where I now currently serve as pastor. My father also was one of the founders of the Nassau Council of Black Clergy and the first African American to serve as the president of the Nassau County Medical Center.

Over the years I had stood by his side in many troubled times. I was just a boy, growing up in New York, and it was long before Dad had gotten involved in government and ministry that took him to town hall meetings, the county seat of government, and even the White House.

While still a youngster, my father lost his secular job and would take me fishing with him every single day except Sunday. I did not realize back then that he had lost his job and that fishing was our only way of getting food. But I sure do appreciate it now as I look at the little faces of my three children.

As I reflect back on that example, I appreciate it because I did not realize then as a child that many boys did not have a father around. The testimony of my father's life and his lasting legacy is real revival in troubled times.

His example of going fishing when he lost his job gives me godly courage not to give up when the troubles of life come my way. That fish fed our family of five a great dinner!

At the time of this writing I am about to release the evangelism team that my father/pastor, my spiritual father in the ministry, started just prior to his being diagnosed with cancer. Even in his troubled times he still wanted to go fishing "spiritually." If he could not physically get up and fish himself he would establish an evangelism team to be fishers of men to win lost souls to Christ.

Our church also is busy planning for our first soul-winning conference. Dad could not take us fishing as he did when I was young, but as he lay in a hospital bed in pain and agony he asked me to go "fishing" with him one more time by becoming his co-pastor. I served as co-pastor in troubled times.

There were several deaths in the church, but we kept the people encouraged in the Lord. I had to preach funerals of longtime members while Dad was in a hospital bed right next door at the church parsonage in brutal pain. We would call the ambulance to rush him back to the hospital. I saw many people healed of all types of diseases as we changed my father's colostomy bag and cared for his wounds after his two surgeries.

I had to move my family out of our two-bedroom apartment into a one-bedroom. At one point I had my wife, my first-born daughter, my son, and my new baby girl—a family of five—all living in a one-bedroom apartment. Thank God five is the number of grace!

God can bring economic, as well as spiritual, revival in troubled times. I went to work. Took care of my responsibilities with the church and visited my father at the hospital in New York City.

During my father's illness, saints from all across the world prayed and believed for his healing. I confessed and stood on God's Word without wavering or any doubt that God would heal my father. People that my father had prayed for before he went into the hospital were being healed from all forms of cancer left and right. Even today I still run into people my father had prayed for who have since received miraculous healing from cancer.

My father never received the physical manifestation of healing, but when he died he was with the Healer Himself, in the arms of Jesus.

CHRIST IS THE LORD OF REVIVAL

Before my father died my wife, Brenda, and I, had our third child: Faith Miranda. We also bought our first house, but Dad never got a chance to see Faith Miranda or visit the house. God did allow my father to witness the ground-breaking to the new addition to the Mount Sinai Baptist Church. The construction will literally doubled the size of our building.

Dad never saw the bulldozers on the site, and he never lived to see the walls erected or the roof put on, but in his wheelchair he saw the ground-breaking and he shoveled the first scoop of dirt. He had the entire church lined up in seven separate lines, representing the seven churches of Asia Minor. The preachers of the gospel and their wives were in the first line, then the deacons and deaconesses in the second, trustees and their wives in the third, and so on with Sunday school teachers, missionaries, music ministry, etc. He made sure everybody turned some dirt in the name of Jesus.

When he was diagnosed with cancer, he came and hugged everyone in the church. He was tired and wanted to go home and be with Jesus, the Lord of revival even in troubled times. I believe he wanted to be in the arms of Jesus, the great Fisher of men's lost souls. In fact, when my father was in the hospital, in his worst condition,

Some folks may have lost loved ones to illness, but healing is still ours. I don't know why everyone does not receive the physical manifestation of healing. But whether or not a saint receives healing on this side of glory or in the arms of Jesus up in heaven, God is still Healer.

He was wounded for our transgressions and bruised for our iniquities. I know that healing is ours. Healing is the children's bread. I thank God for my father's life and the legacy that taught that God can revive, yes even in troubled times. I knew that already, but now I know it at a much deeper level. In the hardest times my entire family got closer to God, even in the pain and the pressure. We walked by faith and not by sight.

Single parent, don't give up. God has revival just for you with your name on it, even in troubled times. You, on the very brink of divorce, don't give up. God has real revival for you, even during this troubling time. Divorced brother or sister, God has not forgotten about you. He will revive you in the midst of your trouble.

Brothers and sisters on the verge of bankruptcy, God stills cares about you and He will revive you right in the very middle of your trouble. God is no respecter of persons, but He is a respecter of the principles of real revival. Get ready to go fishing, my brother and sister. God is going to send real revival in your worst troubled times.

In the midst of their tears, in midst of their fears, revive your work, Lord, in the home, for the church, and throughout the community. Though I walk in the midst of threats, though I walk in the midst of persecution for Christ's sake, though I walk in the midst of trails and tribulations, God will revive me. He will stretch forth His mighty hand against my enemies, and His right hand will rescue me.

17

YOU CAN RUN, BUT YOU CAN'T HIDE - RUN RIGHT INTO THE ARMS OF JESUS

Have you ever run away from God's will for your life? You clearly heard in your heart and understood that God wanted you to be a witness for His glory. But somehow you started running in the opposite direction—away from the presence of the Lord.

Only in His presence will you find fullness of joy and life forevermore. To run from the presence of the Lord is to lose your joy in Him. Why should you lose your joy when you really cannot ever get away from God's presence. Have you ever been like Jonah? God had clearly told Jonah that he was to go to a place called Nineveh and preach the Word to the people concerning God's impending judgment on them. Instead, Jonah ran in the opposite direction. He tried to run away from the presence of the Lord.

You can run, but you can't hide. God is everywhere. He is omnipresent, everywhere at the same time. So instead of running away from the presence of the Lord, we must run right into the arms of Jesus, our wounded Healer.

Jonah tried to get as far as he could from God, but God will never leave you nor forsake you. Jonah tried hiding from God on ship voyage to Tarsus, which was in the completely opposite direction of where God had told him to go. So, God allowed the sea to rage. The other men on the boat heard Jonah confess that he was trying to run from God's call. They knew beyond a shadow of a doubt that he was the cause of their lives being put in jeopardy on the raging sea.

Jonah told them to throw him overboard and they most certainly did. God sent a great fish to literally shallow up Jonah alive. Here he is, a man full of pride and rebellion, in the belly of a fish, probably a whale.

Many of us right now are in the belly of a whale; we have a problem. God dealt with Jonah's tortured soul in the belly of the whale. With seaweed wrapped all around him, he had to live totally emerged in the guts of a great fish. He felt all the billows of God's waters from the sea washing over his soul again and again for three days. It got to the point where Jonah began to die to his selfish philosophy of just "me, myself, and I."

After three days and nights, God caused the great fish to spit up the preacher man. Needless to say, Jonah was ready to get on the ball and go preach to the people of Nineveh—just as God originally had told him. Jonah finally went where God had told him to go in the first place—to preach with the preaching that God bid him.

When the people of Nineveh heard Jonah's message, they immediately repented and God did not destroy them. Jonah was angry with God; he had a major temper tantrum. He could not understand how God could possibly give these awfully sinful people a second chance. He forgot that he had just received a second chance and that he was no better than the people of Nineveh. They both had sinned against God. In fact, Scripture says that all have sinned and fallen short of the glory of God. We all have needed another chance from God at one time or another. If God ever gave us the justice that we really deserve, no one would be saved.

Jonah felt the people of Nineveh were the worst bunch of sinners on the face of the earth. How could God forgive them, Jonah thought, forgetting so soon that God had just forgiven him. God had to take Jonah back to that good ol' school known as the "University of Life." One day as Jonah was resting under a shady plant, God caused the plant to wither up, and Jonah started complying again.

God had to straighten out Jonah by reminding him that just as that plant gave him shade in the heat of the day, God's love and mercy gave the people of Nineveh shade and forgiveness that covered their sins.

Jonah did not want to go to Nineveh for the very same reason many men don't want to do what God says. God is calling men to receive inner healing and essential wholeness in order to minister to men who not only have the same problems, but also different and various problems. God will take us through belly of the whale and the University of Life so we will learn not to be judgmental, but to learn compassion. Jesus, who was buried in a borrowed tomb for three days, rose again. Jonah was in the belly of the great fish for three days and was spat out and given another chance to obey God. Jesus wants to teach men how to be strong men and yet know when and how to share compassion with people who are hurting, just like they were or, in many cases, still are.

You can run, but you can't hide. Instead, run right into the loving, everlasting arms of Jesus. He will teach you how to touch the lives of people bound in sin. As you do, never forget how He delivered you from the belly of the beast.

ACCEPTED IN THE BELOVED

By Arthur L. Mackey, Jr.

We are accepted in the Beloved. 0, 000, yes.
In the arms of Jesus, We are embraced, We are loved.

We are accepted in the Beloved. 0, 000, yes.
In the arms of Jesus, We are embraced, We are loved.

The Father blessed us. Yes, He chose us.
The Father adopted us, because Jesus redeemed us.

We are accepted in the Beloved. 0, 000, yes.
In the arms of Jesus, We are embraced, We are loved.

I am accepted in the Beloved. 0, 000, yes.
In the arms of Jesus, I am embraced, I am loved.

I am accepted in the Beloved. 0, 000, yes.
In the arms of Jesus, I am embraced, I am loved.

The Father blessed me. Yes, He chose me.
The Father adopted me, because Jesus redeemed me.

I am accepted in the Beloved, 0, 000, yes.
In the arms of Jesus,
I am embraced, I am loved.

HEALING IS OURS

By Arthur L. Mackey, Jr.

Healing is ours
0,0,0 healing is ours
I know that healing is ours 0,0,0, healing is ours

He was wounded for our transgressions He was bruised for inequities I know that healing is ours 0,0,0, healing is ours

What ever the case might be.

Healing is ours
0,0,0 healing is ours
I know that healing is ours 0,0,0, healing is ours

The chastisement of our peace was upon Him And with His stripes will are healed I know that healing is ours 0,0,0 healing is ours.

What ever the case might be.

Healing is ours
0,0,0 healing is ours
I know that healing is ours 0,0,0, healing is ours

SOURCE OF INNER HEALING

By Arthur L. Mackey, Jr.

Lead - Holy Spirit breathe on me. Holy Spirit breathe in me.
Holy Spirit, Holy Spirit, breathe through me. For you are my source
of inner healing.

Lead - Holy Spirit breathe on me. Holy Spirit breathe in me.
Holy Spirit, Holy Spirit, breathe through me. For you are my source
of inner healing.

Lead - Come on and restore my soul. Choir - Restore my soul. Lead
- Make me whole.
Choir - Make me whole.
Lead - For you are my source of inner healing.

Lead - Come on and restore my soul. Choir - Restore my soul. Lead
- Make me whole.
Choir - Make me whole.
Lead - For you are my source of inner healing.

Lead - Can you help me, help me say yes.
Choir - Yes.
Lead - Say Yes.
Choir - Yes.
Lead - For You are my source of inner healing.

Lead - Can you help me, help me say yes.
Choir - Yes.
Lead - Say Yes.
Choir - Yes.
Lead - For You are my source of inner healing.

BIBLIOGRAPHY

CHAPTER 1

1.) Sherwood Eliot Wirt, *Jesus Man of Joy*, Thomas Nelson Publishers, Nashville, Tenn., 1991, p. 19.

2.) Dr. Edwin Louis Cole, *On Becoming a Real Man*, Thomas Nelson Publishers, 1992, p. 5.

3.) *When Men Think Private Thoughts*, Gordon MacDonald, Thomas Nelson Publishers, Nashville, Tennessee, 1996, p. 9.

4.) Dr. Martin Luther King Jr., *The Measure of a Man*, Fortress Press, Philadelphia, Penn., 1988, pgs. 54-55.

CHAPTER 2

5.) John L. Mason, *Let Go of Whatever Makes You Stop*, Insight International, Tulsa, Okla., 1994, p.2.

6.) "Rise Up, O Men Of God," William P. Merrill & Aaron Williams, *The New National Baptist Hymnal*, Nashville, Tenn., p. 406.

7.) David D. Gilmore, *Manhood in the Making*, Yale University Press, New Haven & London, 1990, p. 229.

CHAPTER 3

8.) Steve Farrar, *Anchor in Man*, Thomas Nelson, Nashville, 1998 p.93

9.) Josh McDowell, *The Father Connection*, Broadman & Holman Publishers, Nashville, Tenn., 1996 p.4.

10.) Martin Luther King, Jr., *The Measure of A Man*, Fortress Press, Philadelphia, Penn., 1988.

11.) Les Brown, *It's Not Over Until You Win!*, Simon & Schuster, New York, N.Y., p. 23.

CHAPTER 5

12.) Glenn Curtis Frazier Sr., *I Have Heard From the Lord, and Sometimes...God Sounds Like My Wife!*, Treasure House, Shippensburg, Penn., 1994.

13.) Edwin Cole, *Communication, Sex and Money*, Honor Book, Tulsa, Okla., 1987, p. 70.

14.) *Sex 101: Unlocking Hidden Truths about Sex*, Myles Munroe and David Burrows, Pneuma Life Publishing., Lanham, Md., 1999 pgs. 52, 54.

15.) Steve Farrar, *Anchor in Man*, Thomas Nelson, Nashville, 1998 p.7

CHAPTER 7

16.) R.A. Torrey, *How to Bring Men to Christ*, Whitaker House, Springdale, Penn., 1984, p. 100.

CHAPTER 8

17.) Geoff Gorsuch, *Brothers! Calling Men into Vital Relationship*, NavPress, Colorado Springs, Colo., 1994, pgs. 16-17.

CHAPTER 10

18.) Edwin Louis Cole, *Courage: A Book for Champions*, Harrison House, Tulsa, Okla., 1985, p. 98.

19.) William Carr Peel, *What God Does When Men Pray*, NavPress, Colorado Springs, Colo., 1993.

CHAPTER 11

20.) Allen T. Sheffield, *Men to Men*, Zondervan, Grand Rapids, Michigan, 1998, pg.61.

21.) Larry T. Freeman, *Dealing with Stress: A Biblical Approach*, Companion Press, 1991.

ABOUT THE AUTHOR

Rev. Arthur L. Mackey, Jr. is pastor of the Mount Sinai Baptist Church Cathedral in Roosevelt, New York. Rev. Mackey is an anointed preacher and teacher committed to reaching the world with the gospel of Jesus Christ..

He is married to the lovely Brenda Jackson Mackey. They have three children: Yolanda, Jordan, and Faith. Rev. Mackey also is the founder and president of Arthur Mackey Ministries, Visions of Victory Ministries, and Mackey Productions.

He is the author of several books: *The Biblical Principles of Success, Walking Through the Doorways of Destiny, Inner Healing for Men, Inner Healing for Women,* and *Real Revival.* He also has written many songs such as "Source of Inner Healing," "Accepted in the Beloved," "Revive Thy Work," "Break Forth," and "Reaching Generation X."

Rev. Mackey is a graduate of Virginia Union University in Richmond, Virginia, where he majored in religion and philosophy. Rev. Mackey is called of God to motivational ministry that helps broken, battered, and bruised people from all cultures, colors, and creeds in order that they would experience inner healing and real revival.

The Sinner's Prayer

The First Step Toward True Success

Father God, in the mighty, marvelous, and matchless name of Jesus, I come crying before Your eternal throne of grace, realizing that the place where I am right now has become my mourner's bench of sorrow and repentance.

Heavenly Father, I am asking You to forgive me of all my sins, faults, lies, misdirected desires, and shortcomings. Today I accept as an undeniable fact that more than two thousand years ago on Calvary's old rugged cross, Jesus Christ of Nazareth washed away my sins as far as the east is from the west. That is an infinite line that never stops. That is how far my personal, public, and private sins have been thrown away. They now have been literally cast down into the sea of forgetfulness!

I personally proclaim at this very moment that Jesus Christ lived, died, and rose again that I might receive true success called salvation. Today I accept, confess, and believe deeply within that Jesus Christ is the liberating Lord of my life and the satisfying Savior of my soul.

Now, Lord, I ask You to lead, guide, and direct me through the Holy Spirit from one degree of grace unto another. While I am on this journey of new growth, learning, and Christian development, teach me, Heavenly Master, how to walk day by day in the footsteps of Your Son, Jesus Christ. Amen.

Name: _____

Date: _____

To contact Pastor Arthur L. Mackey, Jr. write to:
Pastor Arthur L. Mackey, Jr.
Mt. Sinai Baptist Church Cathedral
243 Rev. Dr. Arthur L. Mackey, Sr. Avenue
Roosevelt, New York 11575
Or visit the website
www.mtsinaibcc.org

Publications by Arthur L. Mackey, Jr.

Books

Inner Healing for Men (soft cover)

Inner Healing for Men (hard cover)

Inner Healing for Men (E-Book)

Inner Healing for Women (soft cover)

Inner Healing for Women (hard cover)

Inner Healing for Women (E-Book)

Real Revival (soft cover)

Real Revival (hard cover)

Real Revival (E-Book)

Reaching Generation X (soft cover)

Reaching Generation X (hard cover)

Reaching Generation X (E-Book)

The Biblical Principles of Success (soft cover)

Walking Through the Doorways of Destiny (soft cover)

Compact Disc (CD)

Real Revival (featuring the songs Revive Thy Work, Breakforth, and Reaching Generation X)

Inner Healing for Men and Women (featuring the songs Source of Inner Healing,

Healing Is Ours, and Accepted in the Beloved)

Printed in the United States
1528300004B/241-264